AN**XL**LIFE
STAYING BIG AT HALF THE SIZE

BY
BIG BOY

CASH MONEY CONTENT

CASH MONEY CONTENT

AN XL LIFE: STAYING BIG AT HALF THE SIZE

Copyright © 2011 by Kurt Alexander

Cash Money Content™ and all associated logos are trademarks of
Cash Money Content LLC.

This work is a memoir. It reflects the author's present recollections of
his experiences over a period of years. Certain names and identifying
characteristics have been changed.

First Hardcover Edition: December 2011

Book Layout: Peng Olaguera/ISPN
Cover Design: Michael Nagin
Cover Photography: Zach Cordner

For further information log onto www.CashMoneyContent.com

Library of Congress Control Number: 2011931191

ISBN: 978-1-936399-21-5 hc
ISBN: 978-1-936399-22-2 ebook

10 9 8 7 6 5 4 3 2 1

Printed in the United States

*This book is dedicated to the most beautiful Angel
to ever walk this earth, my mother, Ida Mae Alexander.
I.L.Y.M.T.A.E.I.T.W. See ya when I get there.*

CONTENTS

PROLOGUE

IF I WAKE UP AND SEE BIGGIE

All I had to do was wake up. Yeah, I'd be in pain. It was surgery, not a pool party. But I'd already had a weight loss surgery—the controversial duodenal switch—to get a handle on the 500-plus pounds I'd topped out at by age 34. I knew I had a high threshold for pain. I wasn't tripping over a little procedure to remove the 40 to 50 pounds of excess skin I'd been left with since the duodenal switch had helped me lose nearly half my body weight.

Sure, I'd been clowning before the surgery: "Well, damn, if I wake up and see Biggie and Tupac, then I know the procedure went wrong."

But nothing was going to go wrong. I was Big Boy. I'd been a player in hip hop radio and culture since 1994. And I was still the force behind the live, weekday morning radio show *Big Boy's Neighborhood*, which had been the number one rated radio show in our timeslot in Los Angeles since 1999.

Lifer that I am, the best part of my success was when the hip hop world I'd loved from the outside as a kid became my world, too. Ice Cube rapped at my birthday party. Will.i.am flew me to Vegas to check out some new tracks. And I'm not saying that like I'm so cool, either. I'm saying that like I was thinking it when it happened: *I can't fucking believe how dope this is!* Just like I know all of you would be thinking too, if it'd been you. That's how I approach my gig—I'm representing my listeners by going to the places they want to go and taking them along for the ride.

At the time of my skin removal operation in December 2006, I was just where I wanted to be. And I had busted my ass for twelve years to get there. I was Big Boy. Some little surgery wasn't going to slow me down.

The plan was to cut open my chest, pull off my skin, remove my nipples and put them on a table until the process was finished up. The surgeon would split me down around my bikini line, remove all that love skin, and then tighten it all up in the middle. At the end, I'd have a thousand stitches. I can see you cringing at that description, but it sounds worse than it was.

I didn't even have to go to the hospital. The whole thing was going down at the Roxbury Institute in Beverly Hills. I'd met my surgeon Dr. Jay Calvert through *The Tyra Banks Show*, which I'd been a guest on following my weight loss surgery. He was the go-to guy for this kind of stuff. You know how it is—people in Beverly Hills have a go-to guy for everything, especially plastic surgery.

Then, I'd go to a fancy medical hotel nearby, where people recovered from nose jobs and surgeries like mine. Dr. Calvert told me that Cedars-Sinai hospital was down the street, almost as a throwaway, he didn't really have to mention it, because we would never need to go there.

After the surgery, I woke up. They had moved me to the medical hotel.

I was lying in bed, relaxing. My fiancée Veronica, who's now my wife, and the nurse were right there with me.

Then, maybe twenty minutes in, it felt like something just hit me. It was a similar feeling to when you get real sick, and it's all over you, and you can't get comfortable. Nausea. Pain. Fever.

"I feel so bad, I feel like I gotta throw up," I said.

Veronica stood at the side of my bed. She looked worried.

"We've got to feed him," the nurse said. "We've got to get some nutrients in him."

Veronica tried to feed me some jello. I was so out of it that it felt like it would not end, like she kept putting the spoon in the cup FOREVER. Once she got the spoon into my mouth, it didn't help.

Things got worse. My eyes rolled back in my head. It was almost like I had to spit or get sick—something—but I couldn't. Nothing would come out. My tongue was hanging out of my mouth, and I was making this noise, like I was gagging.

"Baby, are you okay?" Veronica said.

She and the nurse grabbed either side of me—I was still a big boy—and they did their best to sit me up in bed. They leaned me forward, in case I did vomit. And then, I smelled it: blood. My whole back was nothing but blood from the incisions.

"I'm not feeling right," I said. "I am not feeling right."

And then, I blacked out.

I woke up to chaos in the room.

"What's going on here?" I asked. "What's happening?"

But I couldn't hold on long enough to find out. Just like that, I was out again.

I came to and heard the sound of someone saying, "Take his blood pressure."

It was like there was a fishbowl effect on my vision. I couldn't see the edges of the room, just Veronica and the nurse by my bed. The room was dark beyond them.

"What's going on?" I said. " What's going on?"

And, then, I was out again. They made me inhale some smelling salts.

BOOM! I woke up.

"What's going on?" I said again. "What's going on?"

No matter how many times I asked, no one could say anything. Because no one knew. At one point, Dr. Calvert's assistant was at the foot of the bed. I locked eyes with him. He had this face on him that was just full of fear. That look said it all. They had no idea what was happening or what to do for me.

Okay, I'm fucked up, I thought.

I took that into my next blackout.

While I was out, I saw Biggie. It could have been the drugs. But I saw him. For real. And, right then, I knew it was bad.

Every time I woke up, it got worse. Veronica was crying, just bawling. The doctors were going crazy.

And then, I heard them say, "We've got to take him to Cedars."

The only way I was going to Cedars was if something had gone wrong.

Something went wrong. But what?

I couldn't hold on long enough to find out. I blacked out again.

I came to again, thinking, *Oh my God, I'm dying.*

It hit me. I thought about my choices. *Which way do I want to walk? Do I want to walk through death's door, or do I want to walk through the door to have more days?*

That's how close I was to the white light.

But I was going to fight.

I didn't want to die. For years, I'd had the "it can't happen to me" attitude about what my morbid obesity was doing to my body and my life span. You know what I'm talking about. We've all got that part of our personality that tries to look the other way when we're doing something we know is not good for us. But, finally, I had gotten big enough that I'd been forced to get it: *not only could it happen to me; it was happening to me.* I would die if I didn't lose the weight. And I wanted to live.

So I had gotten the most extreme form of weight loss surgery there was. At 500 plus pounds, I knew I was an extreme case. I had thought all I had to do was wake up from that surgery, too. That procedure was supposed to help me lose weight by restricting my eating through the removal of about eighty percent of my stomach. The surgery would cause my body to malabsorb fat by rerouting a portion of my small intestine. But it had also caused my body to start malabsorbing nutrients and nearly starving itself to death, forcing me to fight back. I had survived swelling, blackouts, seizures, feeling worse than I'd thought a brother could feel. I'd already gotten through all of that.

Now, in just two months, Veronica was about to give birth to our first child.

I needed to live.

So I started talking to myself: "Dude, okay. Come on, dude, don't."

I started saying anything I could hang onto. This was all about me, the real me—Kurt Alexander—fighting for my life. It wasn't Big Boy. It wasn't *Big Boy's Neighborhood*. It wasn't POWER 106 FM. It was me saying, over and over, the God-given name my mom, Ida, had blessed me with: Kurt Alexander, Kurt Alexander, Kurt Alexander. It was me, saying Kurt Alexander's social security number. It was me, naming all my brothers and sisters. It was me, trying to remember my phone number from when I was five years old. It was me, naming Point View and all the streets I lived on when I was a kid.

I was seriously quizzing and testing myself about every little thing I could think of to keep me here. Finally, I just kept saying: "Come on, Kurt, come on, man, please don't do this, don't do this—don't die."

They kept snapping me back to full consciousness using the smelling salts. Only, every time I came to, all the panic going on around me was breaking my concentration. My main goal was to stay alive.

I heard someone say, "We don't have time for the ambulance."

That's bad.

But I blocked it out and kept talking to myself, "Oh my God, dude, you're dying. Fuck, you are dying. This isn't a drug thing or, you know, something where you'll get past it. Kurt, come on, keep fighting, man, please God, please God, please Kurt, fight. Come on."

I heard: "We've got to bring the car around."

I don't remember them moving me, but the next thing I knew, I could feel the lights above me. I felt the wind on my face from how fast the doctors were pushing me in the wheelchair. Then, it got cold and I knew I was outside in an underground parking garage. Somebody was trying to get me up into the car. I slid out of their grasp a little bit, slumped down towards the ground, but then they pushed me into the car. I could feel the seat go back beneath me. Veronica was in the car with me, sitting in the back seat. We were driving, and I was still going in and out of consciousness. She was trying to talk to me, but I couldn't make out what she was saying, just that her voice sounded nervous. I could roll my head over and see her. When I did, she was crying. I just kept hanging on.

Kurt Alexander. Kurt Alexander. Kurt Alexander. God, please, God, please, God, please, God, please.

The car stopped at Cedar's. I couldn't open my eyes. But I could hear the panic in Dr. Calvert's voice, "We have an emergency. Can we get somebody to help us get him out of the car?"

There was a commotion of some sort. My eyes were still closed.

"Could you help us?" Veronica said.

I opened my eyes. Two hospital workers came over and tried to get me out of the car. They must have thought they had a grip on me, but I was dead weight. I collapsed onto the ground. They picked me up. Then the craziest thing went down. It happened to me all the time, in the grocery store, at the movies, out at a club, but I wasn't expecting it to happen to me when I was pulling up to the ER.

"Oh, that's Big Boy," one of the guys said as they got me into a wheelchair.

I was too out of it to acknowledge them the way I usually do with my fans. I was too busy dying.

But they were right. That's who I was, Big Boy of *Big Boy's Neighborhood*. Big Boy of POWER 106 FM. I had gotten to this place in my career by being Big Boy. And I had gotten to this hospital parking lot by denying what so many years of being Big Boy had done to my health.

But I had made it: Big Boy—and Kurt Alexander—were both still alive. We were both going to keep fighting.

AN **XL** LIFE
STAYING BIG AT HALF THE SIZE

1

LITTLE BIG BOY

Even big boys start out little. I didn't stay that way for long, though. Way before I got my MC handle Big Boy, I came into this world as Kurt Alexander, born to Charles and Ida Alexander, on September 8, 1969 in Peoria, Illinois. I'm the second youngest of seven kids: Keith, Charlene, Sheila, Sherrille, Kenneth (who we call Mouse), Kurt (a.k.a. Big, that's me) and Nicole.

We lived in Chicago until I was two or three. Then me, Mom, and my brothers and sisters moved to Los Angeles, sometime in late 1972. My mom was pregnant at the time with my little sister Nicole, who was born in L.A. in January 1973. Mom's brother was already living out there and said to her, "You need to come." So, Mom moved all of us kids out to California. I grew up across the city—South L.A., West L.A. and Culver City. We didn't have any money. We were all over the place, landing wherever Mom could find us an apartment, a motel, or in the worst years, just a place to sleep. Dad stayed behind in Chicago.

I don't know why we up and left like that. I didn't ever ask, maybe because I never had any memories of things being any other way. Now that I'm an adult with kids of my own, I would ask those questions if I could. At the time, I just didn't. I don't think my parents were in the best position as far as their relationship went. Not that I ever heard anything negative about my Dad come out of my Mom's mouth. In fact, I never heard her say anything about him, good or bad, other than the story of how she came home one day to find him in bed with another woman. He got up and broke my Mom's nose. I don't know more than that. I don't even know if that was the out for her. I never cared enough about my Dad to find out any more about what happened between them, or about him.

The next time I heard anything about my Dad, it was 1986. I was in high school. My family and I were going through our second period of what I call the motel slope. Those were several different periods over the years when Mom couldn't afford to keep us in an apartment. So we bounced around to different motels in West L.A. When I heard about my Dad again, we were staying at the Sterns Motel in Culver City. When I got home from school that day, everything seemed normal enough. Mom was waiting for me. She worked the night shift and was usually around when my siblings and I got home from school. She would make us dinner and talk to us about how our days had gone.

The motel room was ugly and cheap, as they always were. Thick curtains with a bold floral pattern closed against the glare of late afternoon sun. The carpet never felt completely clean beneath my bare feet. Mom was sure to keep the two queen-sized beds we shared made up, just to prevent things from getting too crazy in there. Eight of us had to live on top of each other in such a small space.

When I bounced into the room on the tail end of whatever hip hop song I'd been rapping in my head on the walk home, Mom was in the room, wearing her house clothes.

"Hey, Mom," I said.

"Come here, baby," she said.

I went over to her. She gave me one of her big, wet kisses. I leaned against her and felt safe and good, like only my Mom could make me feel.

"Charles passed today," she said.

I knew right away that by *Charles* she meant my Dad. But I didn't sit up like, *Damn, I wish I could have met him.* Or, *Damn, I wish I could have had more time with him.* Or, *Damn, I wish I could have gone back to Chicago to be with him just once.*

None of that.

"What's for dinner?" I asked.

Maybe that sounds cold to you. But anyone who's listened to me on the air knows that I'm not a cold person. I've cried for the loss of friends and acquaintances. I'd probably be more choked up if I heard about the passing of someone I'd flown with on the same airplane— like, *Dude, I was just on a plane with that guy.*

But for my Dad, I had nothing. No feelings at all. Think about it this way: you can't miss something that you never had. I didn't ever have a Dad around; so I didn't know to want him there. If you put down photos of two different gentlemen, I'd have to guess which one was my Dad. Honestly, that fact doesn't bother me. Never has. I might clown on the show about how my Dad left the family, but that's the most I've ever talked about it or even thought about it. Some people might wonder if these jokes are my way of dealing with a deep hidden pain that I'm feeling on the subject. But there's never been a part of me that's wanted to get back at my Dad, or that's felt like my family would have been better off if he'd been around. I turn everything into comedy. My dad is just another source for material. More importantly, I was lucky enough to have the best Mom in the world.

As soon as my Mom told me that my Dad was dead, I was done with the topic. At some point, I learned that he died from prostate cancer, but I can't remember if she told me then, or if I found out later. Just like that, the conversation was over. Mom got up and started putting dinner together for me.

I know some readers will think that moments like these in my childhood made me become what they call an emotional eater who stuffed myself with food to dull the upheaval of my youth. For most of my life, I've fought this idea because I honestly wasn't sad as a kid. And because of this, I assumed that I couldn't have been too emotional about food or anything else. But I've recently come to realize that food was a way for me to handle things that overwhelmed me. I'm sure a lot of you can relate to this, even if you don't want to admit it at first, any more than I did. But look again, and there it is. You very well may have your own ways of comforting yourself, whether they go back to childhood or not. It could be food or alcohol or shopping.

In my world growing up, there were times when food was one of the only things I had control over. No matter what happened, we always ate. Thanks to my Mom, we always ate relatively well.

Food was very important to Mom. I bet a lot of you had mothers who were the same way. She couldn't always give me and my brothers and sisters everything that she wanted to provide for us—but she could do her best to make sure we were never hungry for long. There were times when we ate sugar and syrup sandwiches. There were times when she had to make a pot of beans last. Sometimes we went to bed hungry. Still, more times than not, she found a way to provide for us. And even though my family's relationship to food when I was growing up—and what it did to my weight throughout my life—is something I'm still dealing with, I think fondly of that moment when my Mom made me dinner after telling me my Dad had died. Like so many other meals over the years, it was an expression of pure love.

Besides my Uncle, who convinced my Mom to move in the first place, and whom we never really saw after that, Mom and the seven of us kids were all the family we had in or around Los Angeles. My oldest brother Keith is eight years older than me. Between all of us, we were like Moms and Dads to each other, too. Our family unit was so tight. I won't sit here and say that these were our glory years, with the money problems and all that, but we were happy. We really were.

My Mom was a remarkable woman because, even when things were bad, I never knew it. We were not tearing down money and spending it, but it didn't feel like we were poor or anything like that. I don't know how she managed it. In those early days in Los Angeles, Mom was making enough. We were staying in an apartment, we weren't starving, and we had all the basics. Granted, it was a different time back then. We only had one pair of shoes, a couple pairs of pants—and our socks had holes in them—but everybody was like that. So I didn't feel it. Somehow we managed to survive and, thanks to Mom, even be happy. I've always wanted to be just like her: a strong and loving provider.

Mom worked as a nurse's aid. Then she became a Teamster, working on the line at different Budweiser, Pabst Blue Ribbon and Miller factories. She did her time there until she got up in years. Then she went back into nursing. While she was working at the factories, Mom was on the graveyard shift. We never could afford to have a car in the family; so, for her to be to work at midnight, she would have to get on a bus at eight or nine o'clock at night just to make the bus connections to get where she had to go. When I think about it now, I can't imagine even just seeing a woman waiting on a bus bench at 11:30 pm to go to downtown Los Angeles. But she did it. It's crazy now because, the older I get, the more I realize how scared she must have really been; with seven kids and no man in the house, she had to be the protector and everything else for us. But she never let on that there was anything to fear. We kids knew to look out for one another while she was at work.

Since we never had a car, we were always walking or doing the bus thing. I don't know how she did it, as tired as she must have been, but as early as 1975, when I was in kindergarten, Mom often picked me up after school. When I came shuffling down the steps of my elementary school, carrying my lunch pail, thighs rubbing together in my corduroys, she was there on the sidewalk, right where I knew she would be. Most of the other kids had moms who picked them up in cars. But I didn't care. She was there. That was all that mattered to me. She always had her hands full of grocery bags but she would still bend down to give me one of her big, wet kisses right on the mouth.

"Hi, baby, how was your day?" she would say.

"Good," I would say. "We finger-painted."

"That sounds fun, baby. What did you paint a picture of?"

Then we would take off together down the street, with her carrying those grocery bags with our dinner in them, walking slowly enough so I could keep up. When we would get to Crescent Heights Boulevard, which used to look humungous to me as a little kid, she would stop and make sure I was right behind her. She couldn't hold my hand because of the groceries, so she made sure I was as close to her as I could be.

"Hold the back of my shirt."

I would grab onto her shirt, tight, and make a fist around the fabric. That made me feel safe when the light would change and she would start out into the crosswalk. Across all those lanes of traffic, with the sun in my eyes and the smell of exhaust in my nose, I knew nothing bad could happen to me.

IN 1975, WHEN I WAS FIVE, WE moved to an apartment right near a McDonald's. I can remember those golden arches so clearly, like they were a mother ship calling me home. I don't know what it is, but kids just love Mickey D's. It's like that food is kiddy crack or something. I'll bet it was just the same way for you, too. I know it's that way for my kids now, even though my wife and I try not to let them develop the bad eating habits that I did. It's hard to say no to that shit once it is in you, you know? From day one, Mickey D's and I definitely had a major love affair. Even though I loved my mom's cooking, I always preferred a McDonald's burger to the homemade burgers that Mom made.

My Mom cooked, unlike mothers nowadays who raise their kids on McDonald's. Still, sometimes she would go and buy a bag of McDonald's burgers for all of us. It wasn't an every day thing. It was a treat. For me, it was a big treat. I don't recall my brothers or sisters being as into Mickey D's as I was. But if I got fifty cents or a dollar, I knew where I was going. Mickey D's was cheap enough that I didn't have to wait for Mom to give me the money for it. And, with even a little bit of money, I could just go crazy. It was a short walk across the street to get to my paradise.

I liked to eat, but I never thought much about it until that summer. I was five years old. My three older sisters were visiting some of our relatives in Sacramento. It was a lot quieter around the house while they were gone, but other than that, things didn't seem to change at all. Well, something did change, but I guess I didn't notice too much because the thing that had changed was me.

On the day that my sisters came back, I was so happy to have them at home again that I met them right at the door when they came in. Like I said, my family was always close, and there was never any of that sibling rivalry bullshit between us. They were always real glad to see me and gave me the biggest hugs. It was a crazy scene—their bags piled up by the door, everybody talking at once—all of the Alexanders back together under one roof again.

Then, my sister Sheila stopped short and looked me up and down. I just stood there, smiling at her, not knowing what she was about to say.

"Oh, Kurt, you gained weight," she said.

I looked down. If I had gained weight, I hadn't noticed. I was still the same Kurt that I'd always been. Or at least that's how I felt.

Sheila looked at our other sisters to see what they thought. They nodded their heads in agreement.

"You got fat," my other sister said.

Huh, I'm fat, I thought.

That was the first time in my life that I'd heard somebody call me fat.

It wasn't like hearing I was fat was so painful that I crumbled and ran into a closet and started eating in the dark or anything. I really was a happy kid, even when my family went through hard times financially. And so, as an adult—and even a morbidly obese adult—when I heard the term emotional eater, I always thought, *That was never me.* It's only now, looking back, that I can see that I really was. Food was almost like a security blanket for me. It was the one constant in my life. Happy, sad or bored, food was always there. Even now that I know better, it continues to be a struggle for me not to organize my life around it. You may find that you're the same way. I know it's hard to change your mind-set and your habits, but admitting it's a problem is the first step. Then, it's possible to make healthier choices.

After my sister called me fat for the first time, we started talking about something else, and then, life went on. We continued with whatever we were doing at the time—probably sitting down to a big family dinner, since food was always a major part of our family celebrations.

Being called fat didn't hurt my feelings. Believe me, when you get to be over 500 pounds like I did, you spend some time looking back at moments like this, searching for some clue as to how they might have set off certain behaviors later in life. Whatever it is that plagues us—whether it's eating too much, spending too much or getting married to the wrong people—we know there's something not quite right in our lives. We know that it had to start somewhere. Some people have a clear moment from their childhood that they can point to as the thing that started it all. I don't. Now that I'm starting to come to terms with the fact that I've been an emotional eater my whole life, it seems to me like many different aspects of my childhood contributed to my problematic relationship with food.

It probably helped that Mom was big—not obese, but mommy-fat—and my brothers and sisters were big, too. Not only that, but a lot of the kids I lived near and went to school with were black and Latino, and they were big too. They weren't as big as me but they definitely weren't small. A lot of people in the black and Latino communities can probably relate to this. There isn't the same stigma about being overweight in these cultures; so, it's not something to feel badly about.

That moment with my sisters was the beginning of a pattern of denial regarding my weight that I've had for the rest of my life. Anyone who's struggled with being overweight has gone through it, too. It was like there were these brief moments of clarity, when I—or someone close to me—admitted to the problem. But we never did anything about it. We went right back to overeating. It was like there was no connection between all that eating and the weight gain it caused. My family and I kept looking the other way about my weight for the next three decades.

2

GO TO SCHOOL

I've never been in therapy about all of this stuff. Maybe this is hard to believe, but none of my doctors have ever suggested that it might be a good idea. Recently, my wife and I talked about the possibility with my nutritionist. I'm definitely more open to the idea than I ever was before. But it doesn't take lying on a couch to the tune of three hundred dollars per hour to figure out that there's something psychological behind getting up to 500 pounds. I really don't think it was not having a Dad. It really didn't bother me. You can say that I'm in denial. And maybe I am. Maybe I've got denial so deep that I'm denying that I even have the denial.

I do know there were a lot of factors that contributed to me getting to the weight that I was. I also know that any of us who have struggled to get control over something that's running our lives, like food came to run mine, or who find themselves dealing with anything that's making them feel less than they should, has got to find a way to face up to their behaviors and what caused them. But there's a difference here. I think a lot of people do things because they feel badly about themselves, so it's like a comfort for them. I never felt badly about myself. If anything, I felt better than average. It wasn't like my sisters were teasing me when they called me fat. It was more like they were hugging me and loving me, while they said it. I only remember it so clearly because it was the first time I heard the word "fat" used in relation to me. And it was clear that they—and my mom—loved me anyhow. There was nothing I could do—and no amount of fat I could gain—that would change that.

Mom kept on cooking. I kept on eating.

When I got old enough to come home from school by myself, I found her in the kitchen in her uniform or her house clothes—my mom never really dressed up—making dinner for the eight of us. In our family, it was never, "Fend for yourself tonight." And she didn't just throw together a meal from frozen food and potato chips, either. My mom was from Mississippi. She could cook. No matter how tired she was, she always cooked dinner. It always came with sides. I walked in, sniffing the smell of food in the air.

"I'm hungry, Mom," I might say.

"There's some cookies in the cupboard there."

This response from her was entirely common. She never seemed to worry about ruining my appetite. She knew I'd eat dinner when the time came around. She let me snack on whatever was in the house. Often, this was something unhealthy. Today, my wife and I try to make sure our kids snack on carrot sticks and apples because we don't want them to develop the same bad habits I did. When I was growing up, we had fruit and veggies in the house, too, but that wasn't what I usually picked to eat between meals. Back in the 1970s, your house was probably the same way: full of cookies, potato chips, anything that was cheap and easy and tasted good. Being a fat kid, I was going to feed myself when I was hungry, instead of waiting for someone else to feed me; so Mom taught me my way around a kitchen. I'd make a grilled cheese sandwich, or I'd grub on something greasy and delicious like that if she wasn't around.

While I snacked on cookies, Mom would pull a whole chicken out of the fridge, wrestle it out of its plastic wrap and fry it up whole. And I mean she fried everything in that chicken, too. She would have fried the head and feet if it had come with them still attached. She would put that chicken in a big pan of oil, and it would be bubbling, and there would be grease flying everywhere. I still remember how good it smelled. While the chicken fried, Mom would cook up a pot of red beans and rice that she'd keep on the stove for hours. For the other side, she would chop up some collard greens. Of course, she cooked them with a ham hock for flavor. And fat. That was some soul food alright—good for the soul but bad for the heart.

While Mom cooked, she'd sit down to help me with my homework, which was usually spread out nearby. Mom wasn't the kind of parent who always wanted to check that our homework was right, and she didn't get on us about our grades. She was supportive of everything. But she had an eye on my good stuff and my bad stuff. She just knew. She got some lessons of her own in, too. In between stirring the pots on the stove, she sat down with me while I worked.

"Go to school," she would say, pointing at my books.

I liked to clown Mom to make her laugh, but not when she was talking about something serious. Instead, I would nod my head and get to work.

"Get your education because there will be more opportunities for you to get a good job when you grow up," she liked to continue. "If you don't, doors will slam on you. And there's never going to be anything that somebody is just going to hand to you."

I would look at her sitting there in her uniform, knowing that she had to go to work in a few hours and that she'd be gone all night. She seemed tired and her workday hadn't even started yet. She didn't have to tell me that she wanted better for us kids.

"I love you, baby," she would say.

"Love you too, Mama."

Then she would give me a big wet kiss and push herself up from her chair with a sigh. While I continued my homework, she'd go back into the kitchen to check on dinner.

My mom worked hard. Those graveyard shifts were brutal. Today, I get up early to be on the radio in the morning, and there's some times when I'm tired as hell. But nothing like she must have been. And we had no idea how hard it was for her when we were kids. We were always wandering into her room while she was asleep—not to mention the times when we lived in a motel and she didn't even have her own room.

I remember standing at the side of the bed, looking down on her while she slept.

"Mom, what's for dinner?" I asked.

She stirred on her pillow, opened her eyes, and smiled at me.

"What's that, baby?" she said.

"What's for dinner?" I said. "I'm hungry."

"I'll get up and fix you something," she said.

"I have a project for school, too," I said. "Can you help me?"

"Sure, baby."

She sighed and sat up, stretching her legs over the side of the bed. She never got cross with me, no matter how tired she was. She didn't have the luxury of being able to catch up later, either. She was just robbed of that sleep. I can remember times when I saw my mom cry because she was so tired. I saw it, but I didn't understand it, or all that she did for our family. Not until I got older.

But like I said, even when I was a kid, I knew she was special. She was more than just my Mom. Everybody that grew up around us called her Mom. Everybody loved her. Any kids living around us who were kind of out there or having a hard time were always welcome at our place, even when we didn't have anything. She was so warm and inviting that everybody liked coming over.

And I knew that she really loved me. We all did. She always, always told us that she loved us. She loved us all equally. I never got jealous of my brothers or sisters. But the best moments were when I got to be alone with my mom. One of my favorite memories ever is something she would do, even when I was a grown man. She would be resting, stretched out on the couch, floor, or the bed. When I would come in, she would motion me over to her.

"Hi, baby," she would say.

I was still her baby, no matter how old, or how big, I was.

I would lay my head on her stomach. It was so soft and flopped a little to the side. We'd stay like that for the longest time. And it always felt like the safest, happiest place in the world. Even when I was grown, and I was Big Boy on POWER 106 FM, I would still lay on my mom's stomach and feel that good.

EVEN THOUGH WE WEREN'T EXACTLY LIVING IN the best neighborhoods all of the time, I honestly didn't know how much violence there was when I was really little. I don't remember Mom being scared for us kids when we were out playing or anything like that. But there were some things that were just kind of right in our faces.

When I was eight, there was this 17-year-old kid named Dwayne who lived across the street from us. I really loved this dude because he used to play football with me. And then, one day, I looked out my window, and I saw some guys in suits going into his house. A few minutes later, his mom came out of the house, just screaming. I didn't know what was going on, but I knew it was bad and I kept watching.

Mom went across the street, and when she came back, she was crying.

I almost didn't want to ask what had happened.

"What is it, Mom?" I asked.

She looked at me but didn't say anything right away.

"Come here, baby," she said.

She hugged me tightly, and rocked me back and forth in her arms.

"I'm sorry, baby," she said. "I know he was your friend."

"What happened to Dwayne?" I asked.

"He got murdered," she said.

I started to cry when she told me. I didn't know anyone who had died.

When I went to Dwayne's funeral, it was the first time I saw somebody I knew in a casket. After that, it wasn't like it was natural, but I kind of got used to the idea of death in the way that kids do. I remember thinking: *Oh, Dwayne's in heaven.* And when there were gunshots, I heard them, but I got used to them.

3

THE MOTEL SLOPE

Growing up and moving around a lot was a strange way to live, but that's just how it was. We always seemed to be changing apartments. It wasn't like we were running from anything. Mom didn't drink or smoke; so there was nothing crazy we could blame it on. As hard as she worked, sometimes her income just wasn't consistent enough to keep us in one place for long.

And then, in 1978, when I was nine, we moved into a three-bedroom townhouse. My mom was paying $565 a month. People couldn't understand how she could swing that. Everybody thought we were rich. But, in reality, we weren't making ends meet. We got evicted after a while, and that's when the motel slope started. It was supposed to be temporary, but we were homeless, on and off, for a couple of years after that.

When we moved to the very first motel, after leaving the townhouse, we were only going to be there real quick. We were going to get another apartment. Everything would be better. I trusted my mom, but it was still a weird feeling, going to the motel that first night. I looked around the room, which was small and rundown, and realized that this was our home now.

We must have lived in every motel from West L.A. out to the pier in Santa Monica. I'm not talking about hotels, either. I'm talking about motels that I wouldn't stay in now, even if I broke down on the side of the road. And it wasn't like we had presidential suites. There were eight people living in a single room.

I remember going from one place to the next—and then another place and another. I never felt real stable anywhere because I always knew that, at some point, we'd have to leave. A lot of our stuff had been lost in a fire when I was really young. But what we did have, we put in storage. We carried only our basic necessities in duffel bags and plastic grocery bags. That's just the way we lived.

After a while, Mom couldn't pay the rent on the storage unit. We lost everything. I don't have any baby pictures or anything from childhood. To this day, because of that, I have a real problem with somebody taking something from me, or with losing something that belongs to me. I've lost so much in my life that I won't allow it to happen to me anymore.

During these years, my Mom always tried to stay hopeful. She told us things like, "Mommy's trying to get an apartment. We'll get out of this."

But she also couldn't hide the fact that a lot of things seemed to fall through. There were so many times when she thought she was going to get an apartment. Then there would be some reason why she couldn't. So, instead of moving into the apartment like we had hoped, we had to move across the street to the next motel.

We were constantly packing up our things and moving. Sometimes it was because the motels had rules about how long we could stay. It was usually for a week. Sometimes because we were a family, they'd let us stay longer, but even then, we had to go after a month. We'd hit our time limit and then we'd move across the street. After we'd hit our time limit *there,* we'd go back to the original motel. We got evicted from some motels because we couldn't give them the daily. By this point, my brother Keith was eighteen. He was working, as was my sister Charlene, and my sister Sherrille worked at a drycleaners in those years. Even with their help, Mom just couldn't keep up. She struggled, and she suffered. Once she got behind, there was no catching up.

It was a slippery slope. We were really struggling. I remember there was this one time when Mom couldn't pay the motel bill. I was too young to really understand what was going on, but I knew that she was worried about something. Then, Mom went over to the wall, unplugged Sherrille's ghetto blaster radio, wrapped the cord up, put it in a bag, and got ready to go out the door.

"Mom?" Sherrille said.

"I'm sorry, baby," Mom said.

I could tell that she really was sorry. Mom was always trying to give to us, not take away. None of us really had much of anything. What we did have meant the world to us. That radio was all Sherrille had of her own, and she really enjoyed it. So it was hard for her when Mom had to pawn it. Of course, Sherrille didn't try to stop her or give her attitude about it. All of us loved our Mom too much to do anything that would cause her any more hardship. But I'll never forget the look on Sherrille's face when Mom walked out the door with her radio that day.

"I'll get it back, baby," Mom said.

Sherrille just nodded and watched her go.

Of course, Mom never could get the money together to get the radio back, and the pawnshop ended up selling it.

IT WAS EASY TO GET BEHIND. WE had our daily for the motel but it got expensive. We constantly had to pay that twenty, thirty, forty, fifty bucks, whatever it was to stay in the motel for a night—or whatever the weekly rent was—and so we could never save any money. We didn't have a refrigerator so we had to buy all prepared food, which we could eat right away or keep in coolers. Even now, if I see a big family-sized Styrofoam ice chest, I have a bad reaction. Prepared food is more expensive, so that adds up, too—especially if it spoils and you have to get more. I don't think that helped my weight, either. In the motels, we ate as much as we could. We ate everything because if we didn't eat that chicken, it was going to spoil.

We used to eat on a chair, if there was one, or the bed, or the floor, wherever we could carve out a space. The same thing with sleeping—I slept on the floor for so many years that I went to the doctor one time as a kid and he looked at me funny.

"Where do you sleep?" he asked.

"On the floor," I admitted.

He knew what my answer was going to be before I even said it. He could see that my muscles were unusually flat.

Until the motel years, which started when I was around ten years old, I honestly didn't know how bad we were doing. But when we were living in a motel, I knew that was bad. When we didn't have an address for mail to come to, I knew that was bad. When we didn't have a home phone number, I knew that was bad. I can remember one of the reasons we could not get an apartment was because my Mom didn't have a phone number to put on the application. Nowadays everybody has cell phones and every other kind of technology. But back then, people either had a house phone or they had nothing.

Now that I'm older, I can see how hard this must have been on my Mom. I couldn't imagine my son and daughter being homeless, let alone if I had to look at seven kids and say, "We've got to pack everything up. We've got to move again."

Plus, there were certain schools that we all wanted to go to because we were used to them, and that's where our friends were. So, Mom was always trying to make it so we could get a room close enough to keep us in those schools. That was another battle. Sometimes she didn't have a choice. We had to move across town to start over at a new apartment, or motel, and a new school. When this happened, I never gave Mom a hard time about it. I knew that she had enough to deal with. Even before the motel slope, we moved quite a bit, from apartment to apartment. I remember saying goodbye to my friend Mario and his brother when I was seven and being sad about that, but I kept my feelings hidden. After that, I stopped saying goodbye to my friends. As long as my family was together, I had everything I needed right there with me. When we had to switch schools, I didn't mind being the new kid.

Once I'd gotten over the initial weirdness of living in a motel, it could be like an adventure. When we got to a new place, while Mom was getting us checked in, I would run through the property and get the lay of the land.

In one of the less crappy places, there was a kidney-shaped swimming pool, the water shining bright turquoise in the hot Los Angeles sun. Maybe the concrete patio was cracked and the patio furniture was chained down, but it was a swimming pool. I hurried back to find

Mom in the motel office. When I ran in, she turned from talking to the clerk, who was giving her our room key.

"Mom, we got a swimming pool!" I shouted.

"That's nice, baby," she said.

She always tried to stay positive for us kids, no matter what was going on.

4

DON'T LET THE DEVIL GET YOU

Things got worse for my family before they got better. After we'd been homeless and living in motels for about a year, when I was around eleven, there was a night when my mom couldn't make the daily for a room. And we didn't have a car. So we all slept outside at this open-air mall called Santa Monica Place. When we got there in the early evening, Mom herded my brothers and sisters together onto a bench. Behind us were these fat spiky shrubs and a big fountain. We had all of our belongings in plastic bags, so Mom had us stuff them beneath the benches to keep everything safe. Then, there was nothing to do but sit there and wait until it was time to go to bed. Obviously, we weren't going shopping. Families and young couples strolled through, eating ice cream cones and carrying shopping bags. Then, the crowds thinned out. A young woman came outside and pulled the gate down over the front of a clothing store. One by one, the lights in the shops went off. Everything closed up for the night.

Santa Monica has always had a large homeless population, and so men and women started coming out and getting set up to bed down. A man with a shaggy beard and bare feet came by pushing a shopping cart piled with his belongings.

My Mom had my brother look around, and he was able to find a place where we could all kind of tuck away for the night, have a little shelter, and not feel so exposed. My Mom took all of us over there and we helped her unfold the blankets we had brought with us and put together makeshift beds. Mom laid on the ground, and we all spread out around her. It was cold that night; so we huddled together under our blankets. My brother Mouse and I couldn't sleep, and so we lay together, whispering about what we should do.

"Mom, we can't sleep," I said.

"Alright, baby, you can go walk around," she said. "But stay close and come back soon."

We got up and walked by all of the empty shops, balanced on the edge of the bench that surrounded the fountain. There was nothing really to see; so after a little while, we went back and lay down with everyone else. Even though it was hard to stay warm, and I didn't know any other kids who'd ever been through anything like this, I wasn't scared. It was something that I just knew we had to do. I also knew that we would get through it. Finally, I fell asleep.

Even though we'd slept outside, the next morning was a school day, and so we got up and went. No matter what was going on, we always went to school. Mom headed off to get her paycheck. And then, the next night, we had a motel room. From then on, we always had a roof over our head, even if it was just temporary.

Not long after that, things got bad again; so we went to live at The Sunlight Mission Church in Santa Monica. The way I remember it, they gave people three months to stay there and get back on their feet, but I'm pretty sure that we stayed there way longer than that. Sometimes they'd let us stay in two rooms, but mostly we were all together in one room. We were living in cramped quarters, but we had everything we needed. Plus, the people who ran the place were so nice.

While we were there, we had to go to church three times a week. I didn't really mind. We were raised Baptist, just like a lot of black families. We didn't go to church each and every Sunday, but we were brought up in the church. We knew our Bible, and we were always hit with certain Biblical phrases at home. I didn't think too much about it as a kid. Looking back, I know that our faith must have helped my Mom—and probably us kids, too. At some point, when you feel like you've got nothing, sometimes that faith is all you have.

While we were staying at the mission, we were at church one day, when this lady came up to me. Out of nowhere, it seemed like she appeared in front of me. She looked right at me like she had a message just for me and nobody else.

She held onto my eyes with hers.

"Don't let the devil get you," she said.

And just like that, she walked away.

I didn't know her name and never learned it.

And I never saw her again.

For some reason, that stayed with me. Anytime I was doing something wrong, I'd reflect back on her words. I still think about her often, and I can't tell you how many times I've said that exact same thing. Even today, I tell my crew, "Hey, man, don't let the devil get you."

The time we spent at the mission was an intense period in my life. It left a mark on me. Again, I never got mad at my mom or felt like she'd done something wrong, but I wasn't as happy as I'd been during the months we were living at the motels. When I walked home from school with my friends, I always made a point to keep going past the mission and not even look at it. I didn't want my friends to suspect that I lived there—or I even knew what it was. The building had a big gold cross on it, way up high above the roof. As soon as that came into sight, I got nervous that someone from the mission might see me and say something to me in front of the other kids. I kept right on joking around, like I didn't know the place existed, as we passed beneath the bright blue walls and gold letters that said Sunlight Mission Church. But I couldn't relax until we got to the end of the block. The whole way, my friends and I would clown each other, giving each other playful slaps and pushes, telling jokes, yelling and singing. We were just burning off energy and being happy to be out of school for the day. A few blocks past the mission, my friends turned left to head down the street towards home.

"Bye, Kurt," they yelled.

"Bye," I yelled back.

I stood on the corner, watching them walk away. Then, I turned to the right and started walking in the opposite direction. After a few minutes, I looked over my shoulder. As soon as I was sure that they were out of sight, I doubled back and cut down an alley that ran behind the mission. That way, I knew that nobody could see me. When I got to the mission, I looked both ways, up and down the street, to make sure no one I knew was around. Only then did I duck in the front door.

I knew it could have been worse. At least we weren't starving. We didn't have to steal food just to get by—not that Mom would have stood for that. While we were at the mission, she was the cook for some of the time. She made meals for everyone there. That meant I always had plenty to eat at mealtime. Plus, I was allowed to get my own food during other times of the day, too. Even though I used to have a hard time identifying what was emotional eating and what was not, that was definitely one moment in my life when I can honestly say that I did some emotional eating. Sometimes if there wasn't anything else to do, I'd eat bread or potatoes, or whatever else I could find in the kitchen. And it wasn't like that was my favorite food, or it tasted so good, either. It was a way to make myself feel better and to pass the time. We were cool with the other people who lived at the mission. But I didn't have any friends there. It wasn't like I was going to bring my friends by the mission to hang out. During those times, I became very aware that my situation was different; I had to lie about where I lived, my friends weren't coming over, and my family didn't have a phone.

There were days when I walked home from school by myself. I passed a little Spanish bungalow with a cactus garden in the yard. "Man, I wish I lived there," I said.

I passed a duplex with dark brown aluminum siding and a sagging front porch. "Man, I wish I lived there," I said.

I passed a multi-unit building with salmon pink stucco and old wheezing air conditioners sticking out of half the windows. "Man, I wish I lived there," I said.

That's when it hit me, *I'm homeless.*

I stopped short in the hot, late afternoon glare and looked up and down the street at all the houses. No matter how rundown the houses and buildings were, they were a home; my family didn't have one and wouldn't have one anytime soon.

That's when the charade started. I was still a happy kid, but it was hard not to get worn down by our living circumstances. At the same time, I didn't want to make my Mom feel badly or reveal to anyone that I was anything other than just like them. So I didn't let on, to my Mom, to my brothers and sisters, or to the other kids at school that anything was going on inside of me. And if eating made me feel better, I did that. And if joking made me feel better, I did that too. Mostly, I acted like everything was fine.

5

133 POUNDS

One of my most vivid childhood memories is of a weigh in we did when I was in the fourth grade. There was this male doctor or nurse who made all of us kids line up. One by one, we went up to him. He had us climb onto this big metal scale. When it was my turn and I got onto the scale, the metal arm shot up into the air. He adjusted the arm, sliding the bar back and forth, until it finally leveled out and he could read my weight. He paused for a moment before he read it out loud. He looked at me closely and then shook his head. I felt like I had done something wrong.

"133 pounds," he said.

I didn't know anything about how much a pound was, or how much a regular nine-year-old kid should weigh. But I could tell by his voice, and the way that he said the number, that it was a lot, and that my friends didn't weigh as much as I did.

"We've got to do something about that," he said.

But no one ever did. I just kept getting bigger.

During the '70s, being a really overweight kid was rare. It wasn't like it is now, when childhood obesity is considered a national epidemic and kids are fatter than ever. This was during a time when fourth grade kids were little. To be that big at my age was rare; to

wear an extra large shirt in PE was really unusual. There was probably only one shirt that big for the whole class, and I got it. And it
wasn't like it was hip hop baggy, either, like it was a style thing. It
was a necessity.

At the same time, I think kids nowadays are more conscious of
what they see on TV. It gives them definite ideas about certain ways
they should look and how they should feel about themselves if they
don't look that way. At the time, I don't remember my weight gain
making me feel emotional or unhappy. I mean, the image that we were
looking up to back then was a Jackson 5 album cover with Michael
and the rest of the Jacksons with their big Afros, looking just like us.
It wasn't like I had a body image that I was worried about, or anything
like that. I just knew I was big and that made me different. But different didn't mean bad to me.

My mom reinforced my self-esteem by always being positive and
encouraging me. This was a beautiful way to grow up. The only issue
was, in the case of my weight, I think her unconditional love actually
contributed to the problem. I would never want anyone to think anything about my Mom other than the fact that she was this wonderful
woman who did so much for her family. But it was almost like she
loved me so much that she didn't realize that the way she thought I was
the bomb, no matter how much I weighed, wasn't necessarily good
for my health as a kid. Her love didn't give me good habits for when
I grew up, either.

If you've got bad habits when it comes to eating, they probably
come from when you were little, too. Think about it—if you were
raised at McDonald's, when you're hungry, you're going to go to
McDonald's. If you grew up eating fried chicken, that's what tastes
good. Even if you learn that grilled chicken is healthier, you're not
going to want it. You're going to want fried chicken instead.

It's a complicated issue. I don't know if it's a sign of the times, or
being post-duodenal switch, but I'm real cautious about what I give
my kids to eat. My Mom just wasn't. Partly this was the way that *she*
had been raised to cook and eat, and partly it was because she could
only feed us the food that she had access to and could afford, which
wasn't exactly coming from Whole Foods. So I got the message that it
was okay to eat unhealthy foods. Even now, I look at some kids who

are big and I think, *Whoa, look how big that kid is and how the parent is just feeding him.*

When I was a kid, I don't remember anyone ever reading the ingredients or the calories and thinking about portion size. I don't even know if they were printed on the package. Vitamins weren't even on the radar, at least not where I was growing up. We were coming up in a poor household in a different time. I don't remember a whole lot of broccoli. For vegetables, we had green beans or potatoes with so much butter on them, they weren't good for anything.

But I can't exactly use that as an excuse either because, like I said, as far as morbid obesity in kids went, I was rare. And at some point, I have to acknowledge that there was a lot of food in my house. It was prepared and made available by Mom. It made problems for me then, and these problems only got worse later on. My habit of overeating as a way to feel good and in control was coupled with the fact that, as an adult, I could and did eat as much as I wanted, all of the time.

I think a lot of us grew up this way. And we learned that to eat was to be loved, to be safe, maybe even to show love in return. It was as if by eating all of that food that got set down in front of us, we were showing our appreciation for something we could sense had been hard fought for. And the problem is that, just like everything else we learned back then—how to read, how to tie our shoes—those early lessons have stayed with us. They haven't been good for our health, or for the health of the kids that we're raising now. So we have to start figuring all this out.

Even now that my Mom's passed, when I go to the house in Culver City for Thanksgiving or Christmas, or even just a family dinner on Sunday, there's still a love affair with food in my family. Anyone else would walk in, look at the spread and say, "Dude, this is a lot of food."

It would be wasteful to have so much food, but we always say, "Let me take a plate home." And that's not just in my family, either. I feel like, even nowadays, black families kind of huddle around the family meal, around the holiday dinner. And it shows. Our rates of obesity and heart disease are higher than any other race. It's only getting worse as people are eating more and more synthetic, processed stuff. My Mom may have been loving me too much with food until I was fat;

but at least she was filling me up with her home cooking, which wasn't full of preservatives.

No one is talking about this. There aren't any weight loss books for blacks, except for maybe those by LL Cool J and Janet Jackson. I'm sure they have a lot to offer, but they don't seem to address how real black families are living today. And the same goes for all of the Latinos in my crew. We grow up a certain way. My Mom could make a pot of beans last like my partner DJ Ray's mom, who's Mexican, could make a pot of beans last. A lot of times, we'd eat a whole meal with nothing green in it. That becomes a cycle. We raise our kids the same way; and they become unhealthy, too. It's not out of neglect. It's just a case of not really understanding nutrition like we should. And then, in our neighborhoods, we often don't get the same access to fresh foods that others do. Our neighborhood stores don't always sell the healthiest stuff. So, it's up to us to find the information and the food that we need to get healthy, even if we have to go outside of our comfort zone to do so.

All that love my Mom was giving me may have made me bigger, but it had a very big upside. It made me love myself. That was important because it made me confident. And I let it be known that I could carry my own. I was never someone who was looking for a fight all the time, or someone who was looking for a reputation. But when I look back now, I think that I was probably more ready to fight because I'd gone through some things. Maybe that made me a little more volatile than your average kid. If nothing else, I definitely had the attitude that no one could mess with me, or mess with my family, because that's all I had.

If someone ever thought I was that guy who could be messed with, which happened a few times, I quickly changed their mind: I beat the shit out of them. I did. That's just how it was. I was never a bully. I never went around and jumped anybody—but I never was that guy who'd just sit there and take it. I wasn't looking for trouble. If I felt like you violated or disrespected me, I was going to let you know. And trust me, after I let you know it, you knew forever. By the time I was twelve years old, I had settled enough scores and handled myself well in enough fights that people already knew, "Okay, don't fuck with Kurt."

On top of that, people didn't really tease me because I was always outgoing and self-confident. People wanted to be around me. I had a cool, fun personality and a quick wit. I always wanted to have a good time. Other kids liked that, and I had a lot of friends. If people think I'm crazy or funny now, they couldn't imagine what kind of stuff I did growing up. But it never felt phony like I was just trying to hide something bad I was feeling, or to distract from my family's problems. I've always been that happy guy who wanted to talk to people and get out there and enjoy life.

I was never the big guy who was big because I was a football player. I was fat. But I was never the kid who was hiding out in the corner, or the one that other kids could tease and call a fat ass. I saw it happen to plenty of other kids, but I was never that guy. I remember one time that I was at the Boys Club in Santa Monica. These boys my age had gathered around this one dude. They had him in a corner. They were in a circle around him. At first, I couldn't see what was happening. I could just hear the kids laughing, in a mean way—not like something was funny.

"How'd you like that, fat ass?" one kid said.

Then, I could see that the kids in the circle were picking on this fat dude. They were punking him—pulling his shirt up and slapping his titties.

He was fat, but he wasn't any fatter than me.

When I saw that go down, I was like, *Damn.*

So I made sure no one could ever do that to me. *Never ever.* There's not one person out there that can honestly say, "Man, I punked Big Boy. I pulled his shirt up."

I could be the fattest person in the room—and I usually was—sitting there, talking trash on someone else, just messing with each other back and forth the way kids do. But, no matter what kind of insults were being thrown around, no one ever called me out on my weight.

There was one other thing that no one ever dared talk about, and that was my Mom. I'm sure there's probably somebody out there who listens to me on the air today that has a memory along the lines of, "Man, I said something about Big's Mom one time, and he knocked the shit out of me."

Like I've said, I loved my Mom. That relationship was sacred.

So it wasn't like, because I was fat, I wasn't in the club. I created the club—everyone else wanted to join what I was doing—and so I never felt shut out. Around this time, 1980, when I was in the sixth grade, I got my first girlfriend; so I wasn't having a problem in that area, either. Her name was Bernadette. She had a sister named Gigi. It was very innocent, little pecks on the cheek and that kind of stuff, but, man, did she make me smile. I couldn't wait to go to school because I would get to see Bernadette. At the time, she was staying probably about six blocks away from my family. I used to just ride my bike up and down the street, just up and down the street, in front of her house. I was her man.

Of course, I knew that I was different, but it was almost like that was embraced because of the way I carried myself. I never felt like my weight was a hindrance to my overall life. I never really thought about things that I couldn't do because of my weight. I just found a way to work it out. Usually, that involved making a joke about it while I did.

We did have a lot of fun. It wasn't like today where kids have all kinds of video games and two hundred satellite channels—and that's all they do after school. All we had was ourselves. We were always out and about. We would go outside, make up games, play house. My brother Mouse and I used to play in the backyard. Sometimes our friends were there. Sometimes we played just the two of us. We made up the best stories. We could do anything with our imagination. We turned a flat piece of wood into a car. Or, when we sat down on the bus with our Mom, we would move our hands like we were driving the bus.

Mouse and I spent most of our time being these characters we made up—I was Johnny, and he was Richard. After school, or on the weekends, he came to find me in the house and convinced me to go outside and play with him.

"Let's go play Johnny and Richard," he would say.

"Okay!" I'd yell back, running after him into the yard.

We were just young kids, but when we were Johnny and Richard, we were grown men. They were cops. We loved to drive around on patrol, arresting people. We could sit and play that for hours. The game lasted for years.

My sister Nicole and I used to play a game where we were a country band. And no matter how tough times were, Mom always made sure I had a tape recorder and a microphone because she knew how much I loved it. Nicole and I went into one of the bedrooms away from the other kids. I turned on the tape recorder and we got into character.

"Howdy, Texas Ann," I would say.

"Howdy, Texas Bill," she would say back.

"How 'bout if we sing a new song for all the folks out there at home."

"That sounds real good, pardner."

We sang these country songs that we made up into the recorder and pretended like we were recording an album. And then, when we were done, we switched to another game.

"Well, Texas Ann, tell me about your new album."

That's right—I used to interview her about the album we had just made up. It's crazy because we were just having fun and clowning. I never thought that it would lead to anything, but I guess that's where my interviewing must have started.

Even though I was big, I had gotten into taekwondo when I was ten. I kept it up all through the years. Money was tight, but Mom found a way for me to go to class. Or, we found someone on the block to teach us. Despite my size, I was limber. This is when I learned how to do the splits. That's a skill that came to be much more important to my career than I ever could have imagined. For years, I was always trippin' people out because I didn't have to stretch or anything. I could just go right into a split, like it was nothing.

I also liked to dress up in different costumes and wild outfits. I would take my brother Keith's pants, and would pull them up real high and do different characters in the house for my family. There was this one character named Malvert that I used to do from a movie called *Student Bodies*. It wasn't like I was trying to look like the guy or do the guy. Something about him just stuck with me, so I created this character named Malvert. I used to always go around doing voices and improv. Mom would ask me to do skits. I was always the comic relief in my family.

Mom's favorite was this silly fake language that I made up called Abasar, where I spoke with a really thick accent. It was real fun to fool around with. It had started when I made a joke about the accent of this guy who'd come by to collect our rent. I guess I wanted to lighten the mood for Mom. When I saw how happy it made her, I always used to do that for her.

One day, when I was eleven or twelve years old, I came home to find her in the kitchen, where she was making mac and cheese.

"Hi, baby, what are you doing?" she said.

I started talking in Abasar and waving my arms around until she was laughing so hard. Then, this was the kicker. I made my body all stiff and formal and held out my hand to her in the most proper way possible.

"May I have this dance?" I said in my very dramatic, very fake accent.

She took my hand, and I danced her around the kitchen. While we were slow dancing, I leaned my head down on her shoulder. Then, I did this bit where I fell asleep, and I started snoring. That just tickled her. She was rolling.

I had Mom get me acting books. Like I said, I was real self-confident. I tried everything. Even when I was a kid, I knew I was going to be famous. One time I wrote a check for a million dollars to someone in our family on one of the checks from my mom's checkbook. "That's going to be good some day," I said.

I used to practice signing autographs on any scrap of paper I could find—sheets torn out of my school notebooks, magazines, whatever. I'd write, "Best wishes, Kurt Alexander." That was what the autographs I got from people always seemed to say, "Best wishes." And so, I figured that was how it was done. Once I'd signed my name with a big flourish, I'd hand them out to anyone and everyone—my family members, friends, classmates and neighbors.

And anytime I saw somebody famous—which I didn't see a lot of in South Central, L.A., but when I did—I'd run over and get their autograph. One time, in 1977, when I was eight, I was in the grocery store and I saw this baseball player in his uniform. He was so pro. I couldn't believe it. I ran right up to him.

"Can I get your autograph?" I said.

"Sure," he said.

I handed him a piece of stray paper I found nearby.

"Make it out to Kurt," I said.

The whole time, I was looking at this guy in his uniform like it was unreal. After that, I ran around showing his autograph to people and telling them the whole story. It wasn't until later that I realized he wasn't a professional baseball player. He was no more famous than the person who worked at the sandwich shop across the street. He was just some guy from the neighborhood who was walking around in his uniform after playing weekend softball. That goes to show how innocent I was.

I was obsessed with autographs because I knew I was going to be famous. Everybody around me—my Mom, my family, the cats I hung out with—all knew it, too. Well, sometimes I had to give them a little nudge.

I remember giving a friend an autograph when I was still a kid. "Man, Kurt, what if you make it big some day?" he said.

"No, man—not if—*when*," I said.

I knew. The only thing I had to do was to be a good person, keep my hands clean, try to be righteous, and it would come.

6

MOVING ON UP

I don't know what finally got us over the hump, but in 1980, when I was in sixth grade, we moved out of the motels and into a place in Culver City. It was just an apartment. That meant we could put eight people into two bedrooms. I still slept on the floor, like always, but I didn't care. It was like we'd moved from a shack to a mansion. It was our paradise. We had an address. We had a phone number. We had a home.

After we had got settled, Mom stood in the middle of the living room with a broom in her hand and gathered all of us kids around her. I was sitting on the sidelines, watching.

"Come on, baby," she said to me.

So I joined my brothers and sisters in a circle around her. What with eight of us in the room, we were kind of jostling each other for space. But we were respectful, like she'd taught us to be.

"What's that for?" I asked.

"It's good luck," she said.

And with that, she dropped the broom in the middle of the floor. There wasn't a lot of room for it to fall, but it hit the floor. And she cheered like it was the best thing ever. I figured it was some old Southern tradition. Mom thought it would be good luck, or would ward off evil spirits or something like that.

Well, all I can say is, we were homeless again a few years after that. I was like: *Man, we ain't dropping no more brooms. I don't want to block the blessing, but what is this? I don't think we signed up for this—unless we were supposed to be homeless for even longer, and the lucky broom cut that in half.*

For the time being, our living situation was better, but I had definitely been marked by those hard years. There's no getting around it. My Mom lived the same way she did as a child. She had grown up poor in Jackson, Mississippi, and then in Chicago, Illinois. There were certain memories that haunted her. When she was growing up, her foster parents ate their food from nice dishes, but they fed my mom the scraps in a pie pan. I guess that became a memory she associated with having nothing. We had pie pans in the house, but that's where leftovers were kept. If she ever saw us with one in our hands, she set us straight and went to the cupboard for a plate.

"Don't eat out of that pie pan," she said.

No matter how hard things got for us, Mom wanted to make sure that they didn't seem as bad as they had been when she was growing up. I know how she felt. For me, it was beef stew. No matter how hungry I was, I could never eat it. I guess it was cheap and filling, something Mom could throw into a pot, put everything in there, and it lasted. So it was constant when I was a kid. It just looked like slop to me. For years, I didn't even like steak—not that we had the money to be eating much steak. But beef stew was the worst. My wife brought something like it home one day without thinking twice about it.

"Baby, taste this," she said.

She held out a spoon to me. All it took was one look, and I was done with it.

"No, that's like beef stew," I said.

She had no idea what I was talking about, and I don't know if I did a very good job of explaining, but whatever I was feeling, it was in me deep. That kind of stuff—the things that make you feel different or less than as a kid—tattoos your brain.

I feel the same way about those store-bought prepared chickens. We ate those all the time when we were in the motels because there was no stove for cooking. Even when we got into our own place again, home cooking included a lot of chicken.

"Man, we're eating so much chicken, we're going to fly to school," we said.

Chicken I can still eat; but it reminds me of those days of struggle, especially when I see those store-bought chickens in the silver aluminum pans.

Some other things from back then have stayed with me, too. I'm damn near obsessive about checking the date on the bread, milk, or any food that spoils. When we stayed in the Mission, everything was donated, so everything was day-old, at least. We never knew what we were getting. Even to this day, when I get some bread, if I see that the date is close to expiring, I'll throw it away. In my rational mind, I know that it's not like at midnight on the 23rd, the bread just goes bad. But it doesn't matter. I have to throw it away.

My wife and I live in a nice house now. We've got all of the dishes, silverware, and everything we need. But I go to Costco, and I get paper plates, paper cups and plastic silverware. I prefer to eat that way. I guess it comes from all those years I spent eating out of paper plates when we were living in the motels. Whatever the reason, my wife loves it because she doesn't have to wash the dishes.

The other thing I've noticed is that I use a new bar of soap damn near every day. It's crazy because I'm just coming to grips with this. And I think the reason is that, growing up in the motels, we had those little pink bars of soap, and we all had to share. It never seemed like there was enough to go around. Now, even if I don't use the whole bar, I'll go grab another bar each time I get in the shower. If I open up my bathroom closet, I've probably got 100 bars of soap in there right now.

So, even when our family situation evened out, I don't know that things ever really went back to normal for me. I still felt good about myself and my family. I felt like I was happy most of the time, but I think those early years got inside of me in ways that I couldn't understand at the time. I'm still figuring it out.

Food was always a big part of everything for me. Like I said, I wasn't hiding in the closet, stuffing my face to avoid some deep inner pain. There really was no deep inner pain. Even though some associations and habits have stuck with me, I was and remain a happy person. Hard times can put things in perspective, too. Having been through hard times growing up has kept me from worrying too much about trivial stuff. But, good times or bad, food was always one of my favorite things in the world. And it became my vice, too. I socialized around food. I ate when I was happy, sad, bored—whatever it was— the way that some people smoke or chew gum or complain.

That's why I'm finally starting to see how this unhealthy reliance on food could be another form of emotional eating. Sadness wasn't the only emotional response I could have had to all of the uncertainty that was happening in my life as a kid. It's complicated, and I'm still working it out. But I think that, in order to be healthy, all of us need to start looking at our habits, especially the bad ones, and where they came from. Maybe your living conditions as a child were more stable than mine, but you had trouble in school. Or maybe you just went through a divorce last year, and it's got you smoking, or overeating, or doing other things you know aren't good for you. There's no judgment here. But it's time to get on top of it.

I think the constancy of food in my childhood was a comfort for me because it was one thing I felt like I could count on when every- thing else seemed to be changing around me. No matter what else happened on any given day in my life, food was there for me.

For example, my most vivid memory of my sixth grade gradua- tion, in 1980, has to do with one thing: corn dogs. That's right, it has nothing to do with making it through what were not my best years of school. It has nothing to do with graduating to the next level, or with having the whole summer in front of me. On the last day of school, they served these corn dogs that were each individually wrapped in aluminum foil; and I just cleaned up. All day at school, I went around from person to person.

"Do you want your corn dog?" I asked.

Anyone who didn't want their corn dog gave it to me, and I gath- ered them up in a bag. By the end of the day, I had probably eighteen or twenty corn dogs in two or three different bags. And I knew just what I was going to do, too.

I'm going to take these corn dogs home, I thought. *Oh, heaven.*

I ate some, and then I forgot to bring the bags home at the end of the school day. What's so sad about that story is I can't tell you how many times in my life I have thought about all of those corn dogs that I left behind. And not like, *I can't believe that. How disgusting.* More like, *Damn, I can't believe how many corndogs I accidently left in those bags.*

At forty-one-years-old, I'm still thinking about those corn dogs. Whatever caused me to feel this way about food, there's no way it's healthy. That is how a person ends up being 500 pounds and having weight loss surgery. Even in the sixth grade, I was well on my way.

7

RAPPER'S DELIGHT

If food had always been my number one love (well, number two, after my Mom), it soon got some stiff competition: hip hop. I had heard tapes of one of my cats from New York who was doing stuff that was like real early rap. But then, in 1979, when I was ten years old, I heard the Sugar Hill Gang track "Rapper's Delight," which most people give props to as the first rap song. For me, no question about it, that was the song. And it was the first rap record I ever purchased as a 12-inch single on vinyl.

Just like that, hip hop was everything to me.

Think about it, living where I was in South Central, Los Angeles, that was right where West Coast hip hop was starting just then—1982, 1983—and I was right there on the forefront of it all as it happened. I was in love with this so-called new music.

Right from the start, my boy Trevor and I would be walking to the Boys Club in Santa Monica, and we would rap "Rapper's Delight," with him doing a verse, and then me doing a verse. It made our walk so much faster. Now, rapping this particular song was no joke. It was something like fifteen minutes long. We knew every beat, every break, every rhyme.

I'm sure we didn't look like much, in our clothes that our Mamas scraped together for us, nappy hair, me all fat, him all skinny, tripping up the street together. But we acted the part like we were rocking the mic in the hottest underground hip hop club—never mind that it was another sunny day in Los Angeles and we were walking by the usual apartment complexes, bus stops, and bleached out palm trees. We stopped and waited for the light to change. I busted into a rhyme, bouncing on the balls of my feet, getting worked up, spitting the words out like they were darts.

"She said she's heard stories and she's heard fables that I'm vicious on the mic and the turntables."

I'll be honest with you. I didn't even know what turntables were, but I just liked the way it sounded. Trevor always let me do my other favorite line:

"I said a-hip-hop, the hibbie, the hibbie, to the hip-hip-hop."

Our walk was long enough that we would do the whole song two or three times. We never got tired of it. That was our thing.

From then on, I was crazy about hip hop, just the newness of it, and the sound. It was the music that I loved: N.W.A, Run DMC, Melle Mel of Grandmaster Flash and the Furious 5, who was a true MC. I loved Ice-T. This was even before the mainstream hip hop movie *Beat Street,* which came out in 1984. There was this television show called *Graffiti Rock* that I think only lasted one episode but it had Run DMC on it. I taped it and I used to watch it every day. I can still remember hearing those Run DMC tracks, "It's Like That" and "Sucker M.C.s" for the first time and just loving them. In 1983, there was this documentary called *Breakin' 'n' Enterin'* that had Ice-T in it. And there was another part with these guys who had two turntables; so I finally got to see what they were rapping about in "Rappers Delight."

I spent what little money I had on records. Whatever was the newest thing, I wanted to hear it. The best record stores were Wherehouse on La Brea and Tempo on Crenshaw. This was, of course, before everyone downloaded everything, when there were music stores. Wherehouse and Tempo were where I went to really search for hip hop. Back then, a lot of stuff didn't have to break on radio before someone bought a record. Sometimes I'd just buy whatever stuff was released off of the labels that I liked.

I remember, years later, around 1990, I was in Tempo Records, and I heard this song that just got inside my head. I was flipping through the vinyl, pulling out albums and studying the names of the producers, just like I'd always done. And then, this one song came on, and it was the catchiest thing, ever. I realized why.

Man, that's Rick James that they freaked right there, I thought.

I went up to the clerk with my stack of records in my hand.

"Man, what record is this?" I said.

I stood there, listening hard, and I heard:

"'U Can't Touch This'."

"It's MC Hammer," the clerk said.

"Ah, I met him before," I said. "He did 'Let's Get it Started.'"

"Yeah, this is his new one, 'Can't Touch This.'"

I had met Hammer, back around 1988, at this music conference I used to go to when I was trying to break into the rap game. It was like that back then, exciting, fresh, this feeling that it was all happening around us, and we were there.

It wasn't just about the music, either. I wanted to do it, be a part of it. All of us who got into hip hop formed what was almost a movement. It was like we weren't down with the disco, the soul. This was something that was brand new and it was ours. It wasn't like we had to listen to our parents' music—The Temptations or The Commodores—or something like that anymore. Now we had Kurtis Blow, Run DMC, Melle Mel and the Furious 5. This was ours. This was our Elvis Presley. It was a new sound, and a new energy. We couldn't get enough of it.

And it was almost cooler because people didn't get it. I heard all kinds of trash talk about hip hop from adults and even from other kids:

"Oh, that's not real music."

"Why do you guys wear your clothes like that?"

"Why don't you have shoestrings in your shoes?"

We didn't care. We were rebelling. It was counterculture. And that made it special. We really felt like it was ours.

It was a lifestyle for me, for all of us. I can remember when just sagging our pants was considered strange. Years ago, you could tell who listened to hip hop by the way they looked. If you were wearing your Lee jeans or your Adidas sneakers with no shoestrings or your

Kangol hat, you were probably hip hop. Cats knew you battled rap and they could step to you and challenge you right there to see who was the best rapper. While everybody else was over there, doing the *regular* thing, we were over here, wearing different clothing and living in our own world because we loved it, not knowing that it was going to be the biggest thing in music someday. We were happy to set ourselves apart, no matter the consequences.

I remember getting called into the principal's office after I'd been kicked out of a football game because my homeboy was beat-boxing and I was rapping.

"No rapping on campus," the principal said.

In 1982, when I was thirteen, I got my own turntables, if you can even call them that. Some people probably won't remember this, but back then, we had these stereos that were built into these wooden boxes. The stereo used to be down in the console, and then, the turntable had this arm that used to come up and grab the record. I had a set up like that. I had one record player that was down in the bottom of a case like that, and then, I had another turntable that I sort of balanced up above it. And I would try to mix back and forth with that. I ended up getting a better set up later on, but for years, all my equipment was really piecemeal. My Mom didn't have money to go out and buy me the equipment that I really wanted. She did her best to help me get what she could afford; and so I had to make do with that. I didn't even care, though. I thought I was a pro, and I loved doing it.

DJs had these things called coffins, which hold their turntables, before they came down to the small handled cases that they have now. Back then, cats built their own coffins. So that's what my friend and I did. Of course the coffin we built was not measured properly. Even without equipment in it, it had to weigh 150 pounds. It never moved out of my backyard. But it was our project.

I wanted to DJ everywhere. I didn't care about getting paid. And it wasn't on any big stages, either. These were my outliers years when I put in my ten thousand hours. I was underage. No one had any reason to have heard of me. If I could DJ for free, I'd DJ. If I could announce a party or event, I'd announce. I'd do any club that I could get into, any church function that'd let me in. In high school, it was always the assemblies, basketball games, and parties. I probably would have announced bingo games if there'd been a mic to rock. Whatever I could do, I did, because I loved music so much. As much as I liked going to a club or a concert, or dressing a certain way, when I got into the gang stuff and hustling later on, all I really wanted was to hear that music, play that music, make that music. I loved that music.

Later, in 1986 and 1987, when I was around seventeen or eighteen, I started getting paid to DJ. And by that time, me and my partner DJ Ray, who still works with me at the station today, would get paid fifty bucks. We didn't have a lot of equipment. We'd rent the equipment we needed for thirty dollars and then split the rest of the money, which meant we'd each walk home with ten bucks. It wasn't exactly a winning business proposition, especially because we had to buy a lot of records to DJ. But we loved it.

The more I was around, the more people I started to meet. Once I was DJ'ing all the time, I needed better equipment. I used to rent turntables from Paul Stewart, who went by DJ P. He was always a cool guy—the guy listed as the DJ on the invites for all of the local club nights and shows. And when he started working at the record label, Delicious Vinyl, and started his promotion company, Power Move Promotions, we always hung around at his office. We'd push records for him or do whatever, just to be a part of the movement. And years later, my relationship with Paul would open up some of the most important doors in my life.

It wasn't long before I decided I wanted to be a rapper. I'd been writing since I was a kid, but from when I was fifteen until I was twenty-one or twenty-two, was when I got focused. I really tried to get in and grind with it.

Now this was old school rap. I'm from a school of cats that didn't have explosions and all of those other sound effects to hide behind. It was just the MC, a microphone, and some turntables. That was it. And after all the stuff that's behind the rapper is stripped down, it's really just the voice and the rhymes. The cat on the mic had better have something to say, or at least be entertaining. So I started from that tradition. It meant that I really had to work on my game.

In the beginning, when I got up there, usually no one knew who I was, so I didn't really have anything to prove. I still took the stage like

I did. I strode out under the lights, mic in hand, and worked it from moment one.

"Yo, wha's up?!" I hollered.

From the stage, I could see that people who had been talking to their friends shut their mouths. People who had been turned around, clowning, gave me their full attention. I loved that feeling of making the crowd come round.

Behind me, DJ Ray dropped a record and the beat came up. I could see heads start to bob in the crowd, people nodding, somebody dancing down near the stage.

Okay. So the crowd knows this beat. Now let's have some fun, I thought.

I broke out my rhymes. Sometimes it was stuff I had written ahead at home. Sometimes I freestyled. Sometimes the crowd felt it. Sometimes they didn't. That's how I learned—by doing it. I never had a clue I'd be on the radio some day. Still, even from the beginning, I always knew how to write a rhyme, how to deliver it, how to make sure I had the crowd's attention. I really was doing more rapping than anything else, but I knew how to bring that emceeing thing too. I knew how to rock an audience. I always had a certain kind of energy, and so I was received well, the same way I'm received in radio today, I guess. I always knew how to entertain; I was just performing on a different stage.

I was paying my dues. Eventually it got to the point where I could open the show for bigger acts. At that time, this meant classic L.A. rappers like King Tee, Mixmaster Spade. Of course, they didn't even know who was opening for them. I was just kind of there, rapping a little bit, and they hadn't even arrived at the venue yet. But you couldn't have told me it wasn't the big time.

There were two nights of events—Water the Bush and United Nations—that Ice-T promoted at local clubs in Hollywood. He'd be there with his producer Afrika Islam and his crew—for Rhyme Syndicate Productions—and I'd be watching them from afar, just wishing I could get in on that. It was a real simple stage, but it was deep. A group could really bounce around up there. Plus, the stage was low enough that the crowd could really get up close to the music. The club had these bright balls of light—orange and pink and green—on the front of the stage, making everything look magical.

There were these cats called Uncle Jams Army, who I guess would be considered promoters today. They used to host shows and parties all around the city. I wanted to be a part of those shows so badly, but I was only thirteen. I was too young to go. Roger Clayton from Uncle Jams Army used to date my sister Sheila, and was the first person to give me some really good advice about being a DJ. He was over at my mom's house one day and sat down with me on the couch.

"Man, I want to DJ. What kind of turntables should I buy?" I said.

"Buy some Technics 1200s," he said. "Because if you don't now, you'll buy them at some point. So buy those first."

He was right. As I soon learned, every DJ used Technics 1200 turntables.

Even better, I might have been too young to go to Uncle Jam Army events, but having Roger around meant that I could get closer to what was happening in L.A. hip hop. In 1982 or 1983, when I was thirteen or fourteen years old, Roger came by my house in the van that he used to take groups to and from the club, or to any signings or in-store appearances they had to do before their gig. When I answered the door, he motioned me outside.

"Hey, Kurt," he said. "There's somebody I want you to meet."

"Who is it?" I said.

He didn't say anything. He just walked me out to the parking lot. There in the van, at my house, was Run DMC. They were on their way to a gig. Roger had just brought them by on the way. I couldn't even believe how cool that was, just to come out and meet the guys that I'd heard on the radio doing "Sucker M.C.s."

Oh shit, I thought.

As soon as they left, I couldn't tell enough people that Run-D.M.C had been in front of my apartment. At that moment, I was totally unaware that I'd later be Big Boy of POWER 106 FM and get real cool with Jam Master Jay before he passed on. I had no idea that I was going to get deeper into this world some day. I was just a fan.

Then, once I was old enough to get in on things, there was Diamond Productions, who were humungous and put on shows at spots like Guadalinda's, The Good Life, Unity Brown Rice and BBQ that we always hit. From 1984 to 1986, when I was fifteen through seventeen, I was able to finally get out of the house. There was a whole period where we went to see shows at The Casa and World on Wheels, which was a roller skating rink and Crip-fest around the intersection of Venice and San Vicente in Los Angeles. At that time, rap in L.A. was mostly played on the radio station KDAY. They'd broadcast from Skateland or World on Wheels on Fridays and Saturdays. If we weren't there, we'd listen. The DJs Greg Mack and Russ Parr were our radio heroes.

I saw everybody at World on Wheels—Run D.M.C., N.W.A, LL Cool J, Eric B. and Rakim, Ice-T, King Tee, Doug E. Fresh, the Force MDs, Toddy Tee, and Mixmaster Spade. This was before we got a lot of the East Coast rappers out here, before the West Coast rap scene was all about Death Row Records. There were dudes doing really amazing work. I loved to listen to all those cats, especially King Tee and Mixmaster Spade, rest in peace. Toddy Tee also had a record called "Batterram." Around that time, the dope game in L.A. was crazy, and the LAPD had this battering ram that they would use to crash through the walls of drug houses. Mixmaster Spade also had this rhyme on his track "Genius Is Back" that went, "You spend 300 and make 700 back."

I remember that got my attention, *What is he talking about?*

Well, I soon figured out where it was possible to make that kind of money.

The clubs had a look, a feel, an ambiance. Hip hop in L.A. was mostly black people, but my Latino people were all up in there from the beginning, too, repping hard. Cats like Julio G, Tony G, Kid Frost, Mellow Man Ace and Tony A, just to name a few. On a typical night at World on Wheels, there'd be a thousand teenagers like me. The promoters always had to shut the doors to keep too many people from going in. We'd all be crammed in together, flirting, clowning, freestyling and showing off. There were drugs, but not like how it is now, where you can always smell that sticky green in the air. That's not why the people were there. They were either there for the music or to kill somebody. That's no joke.

Sometimes we didn't get to see the headliner because things got shut down. Either way, there was always guaranteed to be a fight or a shooting. It could be massive. One night, I heard this loud commotion above the throbbing beat of the music and the noise of the kids. It was packed in there, as always, so I couldn't see what was going down. But I could feel this movement in the crowd. Kids tried to push back from the scuffle while remaining close enough to see it happen. The crowd parted and I saw this dude getting his eye dug out with a key.

Oh, shit, I thought.

I was just there for the music, but things could get serious. I got into the habit of checking myself before I stepped out. I had to make sure I was cool:

What color am I wearing?

How many people am I rolling with?

That was during the time when I was trying to rap. So, I also used to go to this thing called BRE, or Black Radio Exclusive. That's the spot where I first met MC Hammer. I saw the most amazing people there—Big Daddy Kane, Russell Simmons, Will Smith. It's crazy because in 1987, when I was around eighteen, I got my picture taken with Will, not knowing what a huge role he'd come to play in my life later on.

During my high school years, there was another crew of promoters called Ultrawave, who were different from Diamond Productions. They would do nights at the Veteran's Memorial Auditorium in Culver City. I wanted to be a part of that so bad. I never got to be and was always a paying spectator, which was great, too. They had that shit on lock.

This whole time, I took whatever gigs I could get. People didn't pay for cats to come rap at their parties if they weren't known. So I got them to have me as a DJ; and they might throw me a little money for that. When my DJ'ing took off, I was like, *Okay, let me DJ on the turntables.* But my rapping aspirations were still there. I threw everything up against the wall. Whatever took off was what I was going to do. But I was still sure I was going to be king cool rap daddy. No one could tell me otherwise.

8

GANGSTA

Music was my life. But around the time that I first got into hip hop, I got mesmerized by gangbanging, too. It wasn't just me, either. Something happened in 1981, the summer between sixth and seventh grade. When I went back to school that fall, I started at a new school, Marina Del Rey Junior High. The ninth graders seemed like full-on gangstas to us. My friends and I all got intrigued by the so-called gangsta life. It got into all of our systems.

Of course, I was aware of gangs before this. Living where I did in Los Angeles at that time, it would have been impossible not to have been, especially as there was an explosion of gangs around this time, 1982–1983, same as there was with hip hop. My eldest brother Keith had kind of dabbled with a little bit of gangster stuff, but not really. And my older brother Mouse had started a little bit before me. But then, all of the sudden, I don't know what it was about that summer, but the number of gangbangers in my neighborhood just blew up. I lived three blocks away from Mar Vista Gardens housing project. Me and my boy Mic Carranza would go to the projects every day. I would see cats with their creased khakis—how clean they were and how all the girls were around them. I idolized that. So all of the kids my age, we all came back to school that year with the gangsta uniform: Dickies or khakis, plaid Pendleton shirts, crisp white T-shirts, house shoes. We even started ironing and all of that, to get the right look.

Of course, just like with hip hop at the time, with gangs, people knew who you were based on what you wore. When you rapped, you looked a certain way. When you skateboarded, you looked a certain way. When you gangbanged, you looked a certain way. So if you put on a pair of Dickeys, or a pair of khakis, you were labeled.

It was the same way with earrings back then. Like, today, I've got both of my ears pierced, and it ain't no big thing. But, growing up, if you had your right ear pierced, you were a Blood. If you had your left ear pierced, you were a Crip. People wouldn't even have to ask you because that was just how it was. When they looked at you, they knew. If gangsters saw a certain earring in a certain ear, they knew that person was cool, or that they had to fuck that person up.

I was all about the look. I would shop at Western Surplus, which was on Western and Manchester Avenues before the Rodney King riot. Or, I would shop out of a catalogue from this store called Hammer and Lewis. If I managed to get any money, that's where I bought my Romeos, Dickies, striped shirts and Pendletons, one piece at a time, until finally, I had everything I needed to complete the look.

It started off as only the wardrobe. Then some of my homeys started getting jumped in. A lot of cats in Culver City were Latino; so they were the Culver City Diablos, the Dukes, the Pee-Wees, and the Culver City Boys. A lot of my black partners went on to become Venice Shoreline Crips. Sho' Line for short.

When I got into that culture, for me, it was like how I am with everything; I'm compulsive, I guess. Once I got started, I really enjoyed it. I liked ironing my red rags and clothes. I loved being around the whole lifestyle. And it wasn't because I liked to party, either. I never sipped beer or smoked bud, or even smoked a cigarette, but I loved just being a part of something. Except for one thing.

I remember, one time, I was walking out of the house, and my Mom saw my outfit. I stopped right before I went out the door. She was sitting there in a chair and just looked at me. She knew exactly what my clothes meant, and didn't condone any of that. She didn't say anything, but she shook her head at me. That just destroyed me. Not enough to go change clothes right then, but enough to where I walked out thinking: *Oh shit, she doesn't approve of this.* Making my Mom happy meant everything to me. That's why I never hit the booze or pot or messed around too bad in school. Sure, my middle school years were crazy. I was just kind of floating through different schools and getting into trouble—slacking off, fighting more, even with knives sometimes, and missing school. One day, I climbed out the window in math class and was absent for over a month. But that only lasted a little bit. And after that, I was back to trying to make her proud, and making sure she didn't find out about the things I did that wouldn't.

At the age of 12 or 13, though, it was really hard to resist this thing that I thought was so cool and that all of my friends were doing. And so, even though I knew Mom didn't approve, I kept dressing like a gangbanger and affiliating with gangs. In 1983 or 1984, after a few years of this, my Mom and I were in a store when these four dudes came up to us. They got right into my face and told me I was flamed up, wearing the wrong shit in the wrong area.

"Oh, Cuz, what's happening, nigga?" one guy said.

"Nothing, man," I said.

"Oh, man, you from over here?" they kept asking.

They wanted to know who I was affiliated with and so on.

Luckily, Mom was in another section of the store. She couldn't see what was happening. She would have been oblivious to what all was going down, but still. I was trying to keep my cool to avoid starting anything that would get her attention. People didn't talk to me like that, but I also knew this was a delicate situation.

"Hey Cuz, we gonna write you a pass because you here with your Mom," the first guy said.

I let out a sigh, but I didn't let them see how relieved I was or show them any reaction at all. Finally, they rolled away. Mom and I went on with what we were doing. I was clear on the fact that I had just been very lucky, that if Mom hadn't been there, I would have been handed my ass. At the same time, I didn't entirely get the real consequences of what could have happened. At that age, I wasn't thinking about the danger I was bringing to myself or my family.

I was never a full-fledged gangsta like those homeys who were kicking it, throwing up signs. I was just affiliated. I didn't buy into the gang mentality at all. I wasn't about to go do something stupid, like jump in the car and go shoot up someone's house, just because everyone else was doing a drive by. Occasionally, I got into one-on-one fights. But that was usually because somebody had started something with me or somebody in my family. If something did need to go down, I didn't need anybody to co-sign for me. I was going to go, to make sure I did it right. Then, they found themselves getting dealt with by me and me alone. I wasn't about to worry about someone because of the color of their rag or whatever.

Not that that stopped me from posturing to my friends about all of the badass stuff I was supposedly doing. All of us kids were that way. We were all saying we'd been in juvenile hall when we hadn't. We all wanted to be in jail. Meanwhile, if someone was like, "I heard you got an A on your test," we'd be like, "No, I didn't."

I didn't exactly have to make up all of my bad behavior, if I'm being totally honest. When I was in Mr. Steinhart's junior history class in 1985, I shifted in my seat and my gun dropped to the floor. It looked so black against the pale linoleum floor.

Oh, shit, I thought.

I looked up to where Mr. Steinhart was at the front of the room. Luckily, he was talking and hadn't noticed anything. This dude, Bill, was sitting next to me; he just stared at my gun lying there. I leaned over to grab it. But I was so big that I was stuck tight in my desk, and I couldn't move fast enough. It was only a matter of time before Mr. Steinhart noticed something happening. I nodded my head at Bill and looked in the direction of my gun.

"Pass me my gun," I whispered. "Pass me my gun."

He was kind of slow on the uptake. I kept waiting for him to yell, "Gun!" But, finally, he picked up my gun and handed it back to me. I was able to get it tucked away before Mr. Steinhart saw anything.

Looking back, it seems pretty stupid. But, like I said, I'm just glad I had the sense not to get messed up in any of the really bad stuff that was going down around me.

My closest call ever was when I was about sixteen years old, I ran into my classmate Jimmy and some other homeys. This was when my family was living at this apartment complex in Culver City called Tara Hill, and Jimmy's girlfriend lived there, too; so he was around a lot.

I was crossing through the courtyard. They were headed towards the parking lot. They were on their way to come up, which was the term we had for making money; I didn't know what they were going to do, but I knew they were going to get some cash, and I was invited.

"Oh, man, what you about to go do?" I asked.

"Come with us, man," Jimmy said.

I didn't have any idea what they were doing, but I thought about going along. I was broke, so I could have used the money from whatever score they had planned. Plus, these were my friends. I knew it'd be a cool thing to do with them. But then, I got this feeling that told me it was a bad move. It was strong enough to trust it.

"Nah, man, I'm cool," I said.

"You sure?" D asked.

They knew I needed to come up, too, and they were offering to take me along. I hesitated. I had this strong feeling that I shouldn't do it.

"Nah, man, go ahead," I said.

Then, when I was going home, I reconsidered.

Damn, I wonder if I should have made that move? I thought.

I saw them the next morning while I was taking my sister Sheila's son to preschool.

"Hey man, did you guys come up last night?" I asked. "How'd that work out for you?"

"Yeah," Jimmy said, dropping his voice and looking around nervously. "We came up last night."

His vibe was shot. I could tell that something wasn't right. So I didn't ask them anything more about it. I got in my car and took my nephew to preschool.

It wasn't until later that I found out what really went down. These dudes had gotten the classifieds the night before. They'd called somebody about a Mazda RX7 he was selling. They went to his house, went out on a test drive with the dude, and ended up dropping the dude around the corner, killing him and taking his car. They killed this dude in the street. His mother heard the gunshots, knew it was her son, ran outside and around the corner, and had to hold her son while he died in her arms. Jimmy was on the run for a while. His girl was pregnant; so when he came to the hospital to see her, the cops got him. They took his baby right out of his hands and arrested him. He got twenty three years to life. The other guy got twenty four years to life. The car they stole was for sale for seven hundred dollars.

This is what they had wanted me to go do. I was broke. I could have been a follower, but I wasn't. I learned something important from that moment in my life. That's when Jimmy sealed his own fate. He and the other dude are still in prison now. There are a few things from this time in my life that I'm not proud of; but I am so glad I never got caught up in anything really, really bad like that.

This all went down in 1988, right around the end of my time at Culver City High School. Things got rough at home again around that time, too. My entire family, except for Charlene, who had gotten married and moved out after high school, had been living at Tara Hill for a few years. So I'd been feeling more stable. Then, when I was seventeen, we had another bout of homelessness; we were back at the motels again. That was rough for me because I was older and had a much clearer understanding of what was going on. I knew just how far we could fall if we weren't able to get into our own place sooner rather than later. Mom kept telling us that we were just waiting on a place to clear. We knew that it was temporary, but our first bout of homelessness was supposed to have been temporary, too, and that ended up lasting over a year. I was nervous. But we didn't really have a choice except to wait it out.

Our problem was the same as always. At the motel, Mom had to pay the daily, and it just drained her savings. She could never catch up. By the time the apartment my mom had her eye on cleared, she had to ask my play-cousin Barry for eight hundred bucks to cover the move-in costs. He gave her the money. To this day, I take care of that dude. He doesn't know what he did for my family.

While all of this was going on, I was doing alright during my final days of high school. I wasn't the class president or anything like that, but it was more because I didn't strive to be. I was probably more popular than the class president anyhow. I was around 300 pounds then, but I never had a problem getting girls. I would be lying if I said, "Man, I could just go get any female." I wasn't as confident as some cats who could just be somewhere and walk straight up to a girl. That probably did have to do with my size. But, for whatever reason, girls wanted to hang around me, and I got with the girls who liked my personality.

There were definitely some things that I was shut out from doing because of my size, like going to amusement parks or wearing certain clothes. I didn't dwell on it, though. I would still pull my shirt off at a party and go jump in the pool.

And I would still eat. I never thought anything of it at the time. Looking back, I can see that there was something compulsive about my love of food. It seemed like there was always a reason to grab a meal or a snack or a taco on the go. If it was Friday night and we were going to the football game, we would stop to get a burger on the way. Or, we'd stop for nachos if it was Saturday night and we were coming home from the club. If it was Sunday afternoon and we were bored, we would go to La Fonds for the biggest burrito ever. Just like I didn't think too much about what my size prevented me from doing, I didn't think too much about how what I did do—eat—was making me even bigger.

9

BECOMING BIG BOY

Every MC needs a handle. DJ Kurt just wasn't going to cut it. When I was first searching out my name, my options were weak. I don't even want to put this out there too much, but everybody in my family had a derogatory name that we all used when we were teasing each other. My sisters called me Roach because my hair was nappy. But I certainly wasn't going to be no DJ Roach.

In 1981 or 1982, when I was around twelve or thirteen years old, and I started clicking up with certain cats, I was really trying to find that gangster name to put on the wall. My brother Mouse, he was Ken Dog at the time. We were young and ignorant. We'd go up to walls and just write on them, right where we lived—with spray paint, marker, whatever, just tagging. I look back sometimes, go over some of those moments from my past and just think, *What was wrong with you?* But there were so many layers to me, and I didn't think it was a big deal at the time.

Anyhow, my brother's tag was Ken Dog. I knew this one big guy whose name was Porky 2. So I started writing Porky 2 on the wall. When I got into DJ'ing more in the early days of high school, I was MC Scratch. MC was for the raps and Scratch was for the DJ. As far as I was concerned, no one could beat that name. I would have dropped the MC long ago, but just imagine Scratch at POWER 106 FM.

Luckily, in 1984, when I was fifteen, I met the man who crowned me Big Boy. At the time, my family was still living at Tara Hill. I went to school with this kid in the complex, Damon, whose Dad was Augie Johnson, a member of the popular disco group Side Effect from back in the 1970s. My brother Keith liked them, and I was up on who they were. One day we were walking home from school, and when we got to the complex, we ran into Augie. Damon introduced me.

"Dad, this is Kurt," Damon said. "He raps."

"Yeah, that's good," Augie said. "I'd like to hear something from you one day."

"Kurt, you know, my Dad was in this band Side Effect," Damon said.

"Oh, Side Effect. Yeah, yeah, I know them," I said.

We kept talking, just about music and rapping and whatever. I could tell that Augie was still this very cool cat. You couldn't sneak up on Aug Dog and have him not be at the top of his game. If he was wearing jeans, they were very nicely creased and hemmed. His dress shoes or tennis shoes were always clean. Or he'd be wearing slacks and a nice loose shirt, with a dope hat.

"Why don't you rap a little something for me?" Augie asked me.

Now, I lived for these moments. I wasn't one of those kids who'd get nervous or be like, "Um, let me just go home and practice up a little."

The world was my stage, if you know what I'm saying. So I was probably like, "I never thought you'd ask."

We were standing there, and I rapped a little something. I could see Augie getting into it.

"Yeah, man, that's real good," he said. "Maybe we can do something, brother."

"All right, cool," I said.

After that, I'd see him around the complex. We got to talking more and more.

Augie used to look at me like I'd already made it.

"Man, you're a star," he always said. "You're going to be a star, brother."

I can't tell you how many times I've heard that from Augie. It wasn't like there was so much negativity from everybody else or anything like that. But Augie was special because he was the one guy in the business who saw something in me and nourished it.

That meant a lot to me. I mean, like I said, I'd always been confident. I'd always just known I was going to be famous some day, but this really made it seem like it was possible. Here was this guy who'd been in a hit group, who was still active in the music business, and *he* thought I had what it took to make it.

Augie was still recording music with Side Effect and doing commercial music, and so he started asking me to write a few things for him. We'd just be goofing and playing around. He'd start feeling it and have me rap something for him. And, just like Mom, he loved the voices and characters and skits that I used to do.

"Man, brother, go ahead and do that thing where you talk like a lady," he'd say.

By always encouraging me to rap and clown around, he built me up.

Yeah, I can do this, I thought.

At that time, Augie was working with Radio DJ Rick Dees, doing a lot of jingles for his top-rated morning radio show on KIIS-FM. Rick had also done a bunch of comedy albums in the mid-80s: *Hurt Me Baby, Make Me Write Bad Checks, Put It Where the Moon Don't Shine* and *I'm Not Crazy*. So then, in 1988, he decided to put together a greatest hits album, which he was calling *The White Album*. It had his hit song from the 1970s, "Disco Duck," which was the first record I ever purchased in my life, on a 45. Plus, he wanted to add a bunch of new material. And he was looking for a rapper. So, one day, I was at home, and I got a phone call. It was Augie.

"Yeah, man you want to make this rap song, brother?" Augie said. "I'm here in the studio with Rick Dees," he said. "We're about to do this."

"Cool," I said.

Augie handed the phone to Rick, and as he did, he said, "You've got to rap right now."

I was about to take a pause; but something inside of me told me to just go. I took the phone and I went to the bathroom because that was the only quiet place in the whole apartment. I just started rapping. I can't remember now if it was something I had written or if I was freestyling. I went for it.

Apparently Rick liked what he heard.

"We've got to bring you to the studio," he said. "I've got something you can get on."

And that was it. Just like that, it was happening.

This is amazing, I thought.

One day around then, Augie and I were hanging out and he just sat there, looking at me for the longest time.

"We've got to change your name," he said. "MC Scratch don't say nothing."

That's when it hit him.

"Man, I'm gonna start calling you Big Boy for real," he said.

"Big Boy?" I said.

"It explodes," he said.

I nodded my head. I was still taking it all in.

"Yeah, you need one of those names where people know exactly who you are and what you do when you walk into a room and say, 'I'm Big Boy,'" he continued.

I thought about that for a second. Like I've said, nobody ever messed with me about my weight. And I think if he had said he was going to call me Lazy Boy or MC Lard Ass, I would have taken issue with that. I was never Fat Boy. Even when the Fat Boys came out in the early 1980s, I remember a few people tried to tease me, but I shut it down real quick.

Some fool would came up to me, "Oh man, are you one of the Fat Boys?"

Man, I hated those motherfuckers—for coming up with that name and the idiots who either thought I was a member or teased me because I looked like I should be. No one was going to be calling me Fat Boy, not even as a joke.

But Big Boy was respectful. Even though it acknowledged my size, it didn't poke fun. So, when Augie presented it to me, I figured I'd run with it, not knowing this would be the name I'd carry with me for the rest of my life and career. At that moment, it just sounded good. Looking back, I'm glad it was Big Boy and not something crazy like Big Pork Chop.

So Augie started calling me Big Boy. And it just took off. The first time I ever met Rick Dees at the studio, Augie introduced me as Big Boy.

Rick looked me up and down and laughed.

"You are a big boy," Rick said.

And I was big. But I was cool with Rick's reaction. It wasn't anything I wasn't used to hearing. And, at that moment, I was all about being in this slick Hollywood recording studio for the first time. I had recorded my own stuff at home but this was next level, with the engineer behind the glass, just like I'd seen on TV. When I stepped into the vocal booth, I put on the oversized headphones. I was amazed when I heard how crisp the playback was. We recorded on a two-inch reel of tape, which they don't use anymore, and I just loved the sound that tape made when it rewound. When I heard it in my headphones, it sounded so beautiful to me. The whole experience was magical. The engineer on the other side of the glass with Augie and Rick Dees said to me through my headphones, "Okay, I think you can do it better, brother. Let's do it again."

Oh, shit, I thought.

I'd seen all of this in the movies, and now I was living it.

And, with that, the engineer started the instrumental track again and I threw myself into my performance. The rap I wrote and recorded for the album was on this song "Good Lovin'," which was a play on the earlier song of the same name. Rick Dees recorded it as Rick Dees and the MDs along with his wife, who was pretending to be a takeoff on sex expert Dr. Ruth (remember, this was the 1980s), under the name of Dr. Rude. I wrote my rap and his wife's rap. Once I got it down, Augie recorded a learner tape, which is like a scratch tape, so Rick could learn the words. Then Rick got ahold of it and made it into more of the parody style he was known for doing. Best of all, right there in the middle of everything, I was rapping:

"Hey Dr. Rude, could you tell me about my lady? The woman is cold, sometimes she's shady."

I loved every minute of that whole experience. I'd made it!

The only problem was that when it came time to print the credits on the Rick Dees album, I wanted my people to know that it was me rapping on the album. And not everyone knew me as Big Boy yet. So

I came up with a solution. On the album sleeve, it read: "Rapped by Kurt 'Big Boy' Alexander."

When I got my copy of the album, I used to just hold it in my hands. I showed it to anyone who would look. You couldn't tell me I didn't make the whole thing.

So, now, I was MC Big Boy. I was a rapper. Even though I had met Rick Dees and had recorded jingles for his show with Augie, I never thought about being on the radio myself. I never walked into the actual radio station and saw him broadcast or anything like that. I was all about rapping. When I thought about my future in relation to Rick Dees it was *maybe one day Rick Dees will play my song.*

I WAS ON MY WAY. AUGIE INTRODUCED me to so much. Not only had he landed me my first rap and brought me into my first studio, but it didn't end there. Around then, Augie and Rick Dees hosted the premiere for this Whoopi Goldberg movie, *Jumpin' Jack Flash.* Augie took me to the premiere with him, and he always treated me like a star. He wanted me to get out and walk the red carpet with him. Of course no one knew who I was. But I got out of the limousine—it was my first ride in a limousine, which was an occasion right there—and walked the walk, just like I was a star. They might not have known who I was, but I'll bet they noticed me, if only for my size. As big as I was, I don't remember feeling self-conscious. I was just excited to be there.

It got even better from there. Rick Dees used to do these concerts at the Gibson Amphitheater. After his release *Rick Dees Greatest Hits (The White Album)* came out, he asked me to come out during his show and rap on "Good Lovin'." I was with it. I picked out a special outfit, which my mom bought for me—light blue stonewashed jeans, and a white V-neck sweater over a light blue shirt. I remember the sweater was snug, but I was sure I was the bomb. This was my first time on a big stage, ready to do it. Not nervous at all.

The whole experience was amazing. Sound check was the first time I had ever stepped out on stage at Universal CityWalk. It was the first time I had ever really seen what backstage was too. I remember being so impressed with how Rick sent people Snookies Cookies to their dressing rooms, and just the way he took care of everyone who was there, including me.

It was a big, well-promoted sellout gala, and Rick and conservative radio personality Wally George were going to have a staged fight that was the culmination of this ongoing feud. I remember that Rick had a stunt man backstage to show him how to deliver the punch.

I had never even been to an amphitheater, let alone performed for six thousand people. I remember peeping through the curtains as the venue filled up. And when I hit the stage, it felt amazing. Afterwards, I was riding a natural high. Young as I was, I made a point to walk through the crowd. Just as I'd hoped, people stopped to give me shout outs, "Hey, you're the guy who was just up there rapping!"

That whole experience was like an opening to a world I'd never seen before.

10

THE HUSTLE

All it took was recording one rap for Rick Dees. I was sure that I was about to hit the big time. That's what I told everybody. I thought my rap career was going to pop. When it didn't, it was hard to take, especially because I had a lot of "almost" moments in those years. I'd get with a management company and they'd tell me they were going to hook me up, Only, the manager wouldn't do anything. Then, someone else would come along and say he was down for me, and it'd be the same thing all over again. I took some hard knocks along the way. But I learned.

After I graduated from Culver City High School, I went to West Los Angeles City College. I took all of my generals, and then I decided that I wanted to go to school for psychology. That was a mess because I'm already a thinker. I started to overanalyze everything. So I had to stop studying psychology. But I really enjoyed learning about it. Like I said, I always had the philosophy in my life that I was going to throw everything up against the wall and see what stuck. College was one of those things I tried.

At the same time, I was still rapping and DJ'ing, just waiting to see what took off first. I didn't have a job, so around this time, I started selling crack cocaine to get by. I'd like to able to say that I didn't know any better at the time. But the truth is that I wasn't stupid. I understood what I was doing was wrong. I talked to myself constantly about it and knew that I should stop. While I was dealing, I tried to have a heart regarding the people I sold to, but that didn't stop me from doing it anyway. I took the easy homeboy route, and I got caught up in the fast money. It wasn't like I was filling out job applications and getting doors shut in my face. I had no choice but to sell drugs to survive. I had seen my Mom work herself so hard. I knew there was integrity in that. But I chose not to live that way.

I made sure Mom never knew I was dealing. If she had, that would have torn her apart. That was not what she taught us kids when we were growing up. I still like to think that Mom raised seven good kids, but I got lost there for a little while. Looking back now, I'm embarrassed by it. I'm not one of those guys who brags about how street he was, even though I could. But it's a part of my life that contributed to who I am today, just like everything else I've done; so I can't act like it never happened.

I had finally saved up enough money to buy my own DJ equipment. I was doing a lot of parties at that time. It came in handy for another reason, too. I was still living at home, and there were times when I took my gear out of the house so Mom would think I was going to go DJ a club or a party. My boy Ray would go put the stuff in his garage. I'd hang out until my pager would go off. Then I'd be out and about, selling crack.

I always heard Mom's voice in my head, especially when I did things I knew she wouldn't have approved of. I still hear my mama in my head, even now, when I make a decision. She was always the person I could talk to about anything and everything. So when there were things I couldn't talk to her about—like me selling crack—I knew I was doing dumb stuff.

I wasn't ever a full-force, full-fledged dope dealer, which would have meant having a whole empire, selling at a high volume, having cats work for me and rolling with more money, cars and influence. I only sold enough to get by because of Mom. I had some friends who could do that stuff right in front of their parents. Not me. If my Mom had ever said, "Baby, go make that money," like some of my friends' moms did, I would have been the biggest crack dealer in the world, or in jail, or dead. But I always checked myself. I knew I wasn't making

Mom proud. I just did little pieces here and there—and I always made sure she never knew.

Since I still lived at home, I had to find another place to cook up the crack, or I would buy it already cooked. I stopped so many times, but selling drugs is almost as addictive as smoking it. The money's just so damn easy. When things happened and I needed cash, it was always in my head that I could just go back to it.

I had a small clientele of people who knew my pager, so I was more of a mobile man as opposed to locking up a corner and standing out there with rocks in my mouth, selling from there. Because I was only dabbling, I didn't have as many risks to get caught doing something I wasn't supposed to be doing. Also, I didn't have a car, so I didn't get pulled over. Still, if I was driving a friend's car, I hated knowing that I was dirty, that I could get pulled over and sent away at any minute for having drugs on me. Fortunately, other than a few parking tickets and citations for driving without insurance, I only had a bunch of near misses. I think it was God's way of telling me: "Don't mess this up. I've got a better plan for you."

On one of my scarier nights on the "job," I was walking to go serve a "customer" on the street in Culver City. I was headed towards this one block called Kinston, which was just horrible for crack. It was known as the crack block, so the cops eventually flushed it. But this was before that. I had three 20 pieces, cut up in plastic, tied up individually. I was carrying them in the rim of the baseball cap I was wearing.

The police pulled damn near up on the curb and jumped out of their car.

"Put your hands up," said the female cop, Susan.

There was a male cop there, too. He knocked the hat off my head, like I was disrespecting him by wearing it in front of him, before he searched me. Susan picked it up off the ground and held it in her hands. The male officer started patting me down.

Oh, fuck, I thought. *Okay, well, I'm about to go do this crack time.*

"Where are you going?" Susan asked me.

I wasn't about to tell them I was going to Kinston.

"I'm on my way over to Ralph's market," I said, pointing to the supermarket that was before the turn off for Kinston.

"Nah, you know you're going to Kinston," she said.

"I'm not going to Kinston," I said. "I'm going to the market."

While we were talking, the male cop was still patting me down, and Susan was running her fingers along the rim of my hat, right where I had put the dope. I tried not to watch what she was doing too closely, so I wouldn't give myself away.

"Yeah, you know what I heard, Kurt?" she said.

"What?" I asked.

"I heard you sell crack," she said.

"Aw, no," I said. "I don't sell crack."

She hit the hat against her hand. I was so nerved up that I was shaking. I couldn't take my eyes off of where her hands were holding onto my hat, but so far, she hadn't found anything. Finally, she gave my hat back to me. I put it back on my head and started walking, as cool as I could be, given everything.

Man, what the hell? I thought.

As soon as they drove away, I yanked the hat off my head and ran my fingers under the band. Sure enough, there was no crack. Then I realized what had happened. When the male cop had snatched my hat off, the crack flew out onto the ground, and somehow, they didn't see it happen. I had gotten lucky. And not just that one time either. I couldn't tell you how many of those stories I have.

I kept on selling, though I had a conscience about it. I couldn't sell drugs and look at people. I tried, but I never felt right about it. One time, I was sitting at a friend's house and somebody wanted to buy something. When I opened up the door and looked, one of the girls was pregnant. I wouldn't sell to her.

I could also turn it off and on. Maybe it was because I was young. I know I couldn't do it now. A good example is the time one of my customers had a problem with something I sold him. I had straight up told him beforehand that I had gotten a bad package.

"Man, this shit isn't good," I had said.

"I'll buy some anyway," he had replied, not caring about the quality.

"If you're going to buy it, I'll give you four for one. Give me twenty bucks, you get four twenty pieces."

That's how bad the shit was, but he knew what he was buying. He went back home. He was smoking with some lady and he called me. I could hear this woman's voice in the background: "Motherfucker. Motherfucker. Let me talk to that motherfucker."

"You knew what you was getting," I said. "I told you."

Again, I heard, "Let me talk to that motherfucker."

"Hey man, don't put her on the phone," I said. "Don't put her on the phone."

He handed her the phone.

"You motherfucker," she said. "You fat motherfucker."

She cursed me out, and then she handed him back the phone.

"Didn't I tell you don't put her on the phone?" I said.

I hung up the phone, went over there, and beat the shit out of him. I didn't think twice about it. I couldn't help myself. I felt really disrespected. But as soon as I cooled down, I checked myself. I was like, *Man, you're doing too much. What the fuck are you turning into?* Even when I was in the game, I could see how doing crack turned people into animals. And right then, I saw how, if I wasn't careful, selling it could turn me into an animal too. I knew I had to take a step back and reevaluate what all of this was doing to me. At that point, I slowed down. I stopped selling as soon as I could, within the year.

WHEN I WAS AROUND TWENTY, I GOT into the phone game, which was called piggybacking. It involved hooking up cell phones on the sly. I was a mastermind at the phone game. Again, I'm not proud of this, but it was better than selling crack and knowing the personal toll the drugs took on people. This was back when a person could get what they called a burnout number. Once I got one of these numbers, I could use it to put you on somebody else's bill. And then, I'd tell you how many months the number would be good for, which meant that you wouldn't get a bill for that whole time. I could charge you something like four to seven hundred dollars for doing this for you. So it was good money for me.

At first, I got into hooking up phones from my friend Scott. I would bring the phones to him so he could hook them up for me. He would charge me. I charged my customers more so I was still making a profit on the deal. But the way I am, I like to learn about whatever it is I'm doing. So, one day when I was getting a phone from Scott, I got curious. After he gave me the phone, I wouldn't leave right away.

"Dude, how do they do this?" I asked him.

He sidestepped the question and sent me on my way. He never wanted to tell me the secret to how the phones worked. Then, one time my phone went down; so I had to bring it back to Scott to hook it up again. I really wanted to know how it worked, but, still, he wouldn't tell me the trick. I kept pushing. Finally, he caved.

"Well, just go over to Gono," he said. "That's the guy that does it."

So then I become cool with Gono, and he started showing me a few little things. I wanted to know more. I wanted to become a phone man, too. Gono could tell I really wanted to learn. He started showing me the computer he used and the electronic serial number finder he used to grab the ESN numbers from phones. That was good, but I still wanted to know more and more, until finally, I would know the whole game inside and out like him.

That's how I am. I had to become a boss in that shit, as opposed to going and just having him turn the phones on for me. Gono was a computer guy. He was the first one to set me up with my own computer and equipment.

"This is what you do," he said, showing me as he typed on his computer.

Before long, I had a computer, I had my own ESN finder, which located the burnout numbers, and I had all the cables and everything else I needed to make it all happen. Right there, I had the makings for a whole empire.

Once I was set up, I went to a hot spot like the airport. I sat there with my equipment, and when peopled walked by me, I grabbed their cell phone and ESN numbers. Then I took that information home, hooked my customer's phone number up to my computer, erased the original ESN number that was on there, put the borrowed ESN number in and put my customer's phone number in. I did that for probably two years. I used to hook up everyone's phones in the hip hop game: Fat Joe, Warren G, all the guys in The Pharcyde, Ol' Dirty Bastard from The Wu-Tang Clan, Tupac. I was the hot phone man.

My other thing was credit cards. I had this guy that provided me with valid credit card numbers. And then with a credit card reader, so I could take any card that had a strip, and put it in this reader to see what the strip number of that credit card was. Then, I could take one of my cards, which I got from a mailman who gave them to me in exchange for crack, remove its strip number and replace it with the valid number I'd been given, along with the expiration date from that card. When my cards were used, the machine read it for the other stripped card's account holder and credit limit. This was good, easy money. Like the phones, I felt better about doing it than selling drugs.

Not that there weren't risks, of course. My boy Gono got arrested for another crime that didn't involve the phones. He's been in prison for the last sixteen years. He should probably be home about a year or two from now. That's a long stretch. Just like he took care of me before, I've been taking care of him ever since he's been in prison, filling his commissary and doing whatever I can for him to make his life easier.

I think a lot about how it could have just as easily been me who went to jail. Part of it was good fortune; part of it was good sense, like how, for whatever reason, I decided not to go with my friend Jimmy that night that he and our friends came up. If I had, I could have been involved in all that bad news with the car and the gun and the trouble that came with it. I'd also have to live with a man's blood on my hands.

I've said it again and again to the cats I know, "Sometimes in your life, you come to a blank page in your book. This is you writing your page." Whatever you decide to do in that moment, or write on that page, it could determine what's in the next few chapters, or even the rest of the book. And that's something you've got to take responsibility for—your choices and the consequences they lead to in your life. Well, I got a lesson right around then. I knew I wasn't living right, and like I said, I didn't like doing things that I had to keep from my Mom. Yet I kept hustling because I was unemployed. I wasn't writing a good page, even though I was a good hustler and being as careful as possible.

I was at a crossroads. I knew I wanted more out of life. My friend Ken, who was living in my mom's garage at the time, was going through a similar situation. I had known Ken for probably eight years, but I didn't know much about his story. But one day, we were hanging out in my backyard, and he started telling me how scattered his family was, how he still had occasional conversations with his Mom and his Grandma. Then, somehow, we got on the subject of death.

"Man, if I were to die, nobody would bury me," he said. "I would become a ward of the state. They've been taking care of me my whole life."

I looked at him and thought about how lucky I was to have the family I did.

"If anything happened to you, I'd bury you," I said.

Later that night, we went to a party, and it got crazy. Things weren't normally like this, but on that particular evening, the spot was just chaos. As we were leaving, somebody talked shit to one of my guys. I didn't hear exactly what was said because I was already out the door. Apparently, things got heated. We went out to the car and were about to leave. Then, someone mentioned that we had a 12-gauge shotgun in the car. I don't know why we brought the gun along. I, for one, had never touched a 12-gauge in my life. We were all worked up, and one of my guys was holding the shotgun's pistol grip.

"Got the strap?" Ken said.

My guy handed it to Ken, so Ken could go back into the party with the gun if he wanted to. I was telling Ken to give the gun back to the guy who'd brought it and let him deal with it. But Ken didn't listen. He put the gun in his waist, parallel to his body. Right when he zipped up his jacket, the gun went off. I could tell just by looking at his eyes that he had shot himself. The bullet had blown out the main artery in his leg. He started hopping around on one foot. Then, blood started coming out the bottom of his Levis and pooling around his shoes. He fell to the ground.

We knew that Ken was on parole. We also knew that one of the terms of his parole was that he couldn't be near any firearms. So we got rid of the gun. This was before everybody had cell phones, so somebody had to run to a nearby house to call 911. Ken was on the ground, whimpering like a dog, and I could see that he was dying. It was too much. I couldn't stand it, and I had to walk away. I'm not proud of this, but I damn near left him on the street because I couldn't handle any of it—the blood, the fact that Ken was dying. Everybody in our crew had a moment that night where they had to walk away and calm themselves down. That was rough.

Finally, the paramedics got there. I leaned down over Ken.

"You're going to make it," I said optimistically.

Ken got taken away in an ambulance. The detectives had the rest of us go down to the police station for questioning. We had made up a story together, so that none of us would say anything that suggested Ken had violated his parole.

One of the detectives took me into a room. I told him how we heard the shot from across the street, Ken was hit, and he fell down. The detective let me finish.

"That's your statement?" he said. "He got shot from across the street?"

"Yeah," I said.

"Okay," he said.

He walked over to a cabinet and dug around inside. Then, he turned around and showed me the casings from a sawed off shotgun bullet. As he did, he told me that the casing only travels about 12 inches when a bullet is fired.

"We found this in your friend's pant leg," he said.

Damn, I thought.

"Do you know what this is?" he said, holding up a pair of boxers with blood on them. I could see that the bullet had blown a hole through them when he accidentally shot himself.

"Either your friend shot himself, or you shot your friend," the detective said.

That scared the shit out of me, but I was still trying to hold onto my statement out of loyalty to Ken. The detective had told me that Ken was going to make it, and I didn't want him to have to go back to prison.

"So that's what you're going with?" the detective said.

"Yeah," I said.

He left me alone. I waited and waited. Finally, the detective came back.

"How's Ken doing?" I asked.

"Your friend died," he said.

Then he shut the door and walked out.

That shocked me into turning my life around. *You've got to get your shit together,* I thought. As far as I was concerned, Ken had just paid the tuition into the school of experience for me. Now I was the one who had to learn the lesson. There had to be some reason why I was always able to escape the bullet or the jail time. I tried to honor Ken by burying him, like I had promised, but when Mom got in touch with the morgue, they wouldn't release the body to us because we weren't members of his family. We did make sure there was a memorial. I knew it was up to me to honor the blessings I had received by writing the next page in my life in a big way. And the right way.

11

MY FIRST PASSPORT

By the early 1990s, I knew it was time for a change, but I didn't know what that would look like. As I mentioned, I was always cool with Los Angeles promoter Paul Stewart, a.k.a DJ P, he was responsible for a lot of great hip hop music at that time. He had this house in the Hollywood area and everybody came through. He was one of those guys that believed in local artists. So he helped them how he could, including getting a bunch of them great deals through Tommy Boy. He's the one who got House of Pain and Coolio their deals. He's the one who blew up Naughty by Nature, too.

People always talk about Barry Gordy and Motown; but I feel like Paul was a major figure like that for hip hop music in Los Angeles. I didn't realize how big his influence was going to be at the time. Since I'd been a teenager, I'd rented my DJ equipment from him. By the time I was in my 20s, we had years of friendship under our belt already. Plus, I just liked hanging out and hearing the music. I met a lot of cats through Paul too. The first time I met will.i.am, back when he was a solo rapper, long before the Black Eyed Peas, was at a Paul Stewart Showcase. Same thing with the Boo-Yaa T.R.I.B.E. and Cypress Hill. I remember Everlast sleeping at Paul's house. And DJ Muggs from Cypress Hill. They were pretty much roommates.

Once, I happened to visit Paul when Cypress Hill had a record coming out on Columbia. I was with my boy Ray, who I started DJ'ing with as a teenager and who still works with me at POWER 106 FM now.

"Can you go pass out flyers?" Paul asked us.

We were always down to help Paul. He gave us a copy of the record to listen to, which was for their song "The Phuncky Feel One." The B-side was "I Could Just Kill a Man," which became a huge hit for them. From the first time we heard it, we were full-on obsessed. We became like *the* Cypress Hill fans. I had this Cypress Hill hat that I used to wear when Ray and I would go out to the clubs. When we got to the entrance, I would pull the door guy aside.

"Hey, that's DJ Ray from Cypress Hill," I would say.

The guy would look over at Ray and nod us in. Once they let us into the club, people would point and whisper, thinking we were in the group. Ray and I would just laugh.

I remember, years later, telling that story to B-Real from Cypress Hill many times. It always got him rolling.

Eventually, Paul started managing this group The Pharcyde and signed them to Delicious Vinyl. That ended up parlaying into a job for me. They went to play a show at the Wetlands in New York and got into some trouble at the club. They weren't the kind of guys to breed that stuff. The Pharcyde weren't offensive guys at all. But they didn't have proper security. One time, these wild guys went through the club just kind of hitting people for no reason; and some of the members of the group got beat up. Paul realized the band needed some security to look out for them. Since Paul and their other managers knew me, they also knew that I had a martial arts background. I was good with my hands and had a level head. Sometimes security can escalate a situation by pushing people and acting like knuckleheads. They don't know how to diffuse it instead. Paul knew that I did.

I was already on good terms with the guys in the group, both from seeing them at shows and from Paul. Every time I'd see the guys around, even just briefly, it'd always be, "Hey, what's up, man?"

Then, once Paul was talking to me about being their security guard, he arranged my initial meeting with them. It was just like hanging out with any of my friends, really. I remember walking in, going right up to them, and it felt like we had known each other for years.

"Hey, what's up, Romye, what's up?" I said.

He was already friendly and warm from knowing me through Paul.

It was pretty much a done deal. We took off from there. The band's management, which also included a guy named Deon "Suave" Green, decided that they wanted to take me out on the road to keep an eye on the band, along with another friend of mine named Sylvester Wilson. This was in 1992, and I was about twenty-one. I was glad for the work, but I didn't think about it in terms of having a guard car and looking out for somebody's life or anything like that. It was more so that I was disciplined. I had a philosophy of let's be defensive, as opposed to offensive. I had a way of not getting guys into trouble, of just getting my crew in and out, wherever they needed to be.

That gig changed everything for me. I had already kind of washed my hands of a lot of the hustler stuff I was doing. And then, I started traveling on the road and seeing different things. I got a passport and my whole world just opened up.

Some of the first gigs I ever traveled to with the band were in San Diego. My friend William "Fuzzy Fantabulous" West, who still works with me at the station, came along. He had done sound for Paul Stewart's showcases. So, when The Pharcyde went out on the road, they hired Fuzzy as their sound person. Before we left for the first show, we were all at Pharcyde Manor, where a bunch of the group lived together in L.A. Some of them were out on the porch smoking when Fuzzy's Mom dropped him off out front. Fuzzy was an only child who literally grew up in church with his Mom and Grandmother because they both worked for the church. So Fuzzy's Mom pulled up out front and rolled down her window. She took one look at the scene, saw what was going on and started yelling out the window.

"Are they smoking dope?" she shouted. "Are they smoking dope?"

Fuzzy didn't say anything. He just got out of the car and grabbed his bag from the back seat as quickly as he could.

"Bye, Mom!" he called out as he ran up to the house.

To this day, that's still a joke between Fuzz and I: "Are they smoking dope?"

As soon as she drove away, we were all rolling.

That first trip was only a few hours from Los Angeles, but it seemed so far to me. Since moving to LA, I had never been out of the city. So that was amazing, just to be able to travel. It was all new and exciting, riding on the bus with the group, pulling up to the club, hanging out backstage, watching them perform. The whole thing was cool. And I was in it. I remember just thinking: *Man, I'm in San Diego this weekend.*

The next weekend, it was San Francisco. And it was wild to see people screaming—I mean just *screaming*—for their debut record, *Bizarre Ride II the Pharcyde,* which they had just put out. I was with the group when their first single, "Ya Mama," broke. This was just as *Bizarre Ride* hit, right before their second single "Pass Me By," was blowing up, there was this great buzz building around them.

It got even better. Our first tour was with Ice Cube. I mean this was N.W.A.'s *Straight Outta Compton* Ice Cube. He had been there right from the beginning when I was getting into hip hop. I could remember seeing him around and meeting him—not that he would have remembered me. I was a huge fan. So it was amazing to be traveling with him. I remember, one day, we were out on the road, when I went to Taco Bell for everyone and asked what Cube wanted. There I was, getting food for Ice Cube. When I got back to the hotel, I knocked on his door, not even believing that Ice Cube was about to answer. He did, and I handed him his burritos.

"Thank you," he said.

It was just a food run, but that was a crazy moment for me because I respected Cube so much.

Not only was it great to meet Ice Cube, I learned a lot about being a bodyguard from his crew, just by watching the way he moved his group, The Lynch Mob. He was already popular at that point. He had his wife Kim on the road with him. I noticed how he always sort of separated himself from the craziness of the whole scene. His room was always at a different hotel, or on a different floor, and he didn't get tangled up in the bullshit. That tattooed itself on my brain and was a good lesson for me years later when I was traveling with my own crew for POWER 106 FM. I learned that you can't party within the party. You can host and have fun, but if you want to have longevity and a good life, you've got to be mindful. I just celebrated seventeen years in the business—not because I'm slick—it's because I know what I've got and I take care of it. A lot of that I got from Ice Cube, way back in those early days with The Pharcyde.

I learned to always be aware of the last song in the headliner's set, so I was already getting in place before they even got offstage. And then, I was already thinking of how to get the guys out of the building, how to situate and organize the guys at the hotel.

I learned the rules that I needed to lay down for the dudes:

"No girls upstairs."

"No pictures in the room."

"No autographs on hotel stationery."

I wanted to make sure that no outsiders were with the band. I didn't want any evidence that outsiders had been with the band. I know that seems like the whole point of being a rapper—right?—getting girls and partying in your hotel room. But it's a huge safety concern. When you're on the road, your room is your house. You've got to be more than careful about who you let into your circle. It's so much worse now, but even back then, we never knew when somebody wanted to get next to the group for the wrong reasons. I wanted to protect my guys. I can't say they listened one hundred percent of the time, but they understood that it was for their own safety.

I also knew how to respect codes. When I got to certain places, I would ask a local, "Hey man, what's the tick word here?" By that, I meant any words that might upset someone in a particular city or make him want to fight. Like I could sit down here in Los Angeles and say, "Yeah, DJ Ray, that's my folks" and, in the Bay area, I could say, "That's my folks." I go somewhere else, like Chicago, I say "folks," I could get killed. There were members of the Gangster Disciples in Chicago who called themselves Folks. Or in the Bay Area, they say "blood" a lot, "Oh, yeah, man, that's my blood." Or "Hey, what's up blood, you got a cigarette?" It doesn't mean the same thing that it does in Los Angeles. Back then, there were certain words that were like triggers, those words weren't universal.

I was pretty much on point with a lot of stuff. I wasn't oblivious to the fact that anything could happen, but I was prepared enough not to be scared. Not that those guys of Pharcyde were any trouble. They understood the bigger picture. They weren't tour sluts. Their thing was getting on the bus and smoking weed—and they just loved to perform. Even after they'd done a full set for a packed crowd earlier in the night, they'd get together in circles and freestyle. They were great dudes to hang around with. They never treated me like just a bodyguard. I learned a lot from them.

When I became a bodyguard, I was more infatuated with the music and the scene than anything else. I enjoyed the road, but that was mostly because I had the right guys out there with me. It was still all about the music for me. Doing security was just one more job to add to the mix. Rapping was still my main thing. I even got to rhyme on The Pharcyde's album, *Last Cab in California*. The song was called "The Hustle" and it explained my drug dealing days—how that had been my hustle—but I was able to get away from it. Sometimes, if Fat Lip couldn't make a gig, I got to get up and rap his parts. So I never let that go as my main thing.

Sometimes I got to play road manager, too. Suave was the road manager, and he was great. But there were times when he couldn't make it. I would road manage, and I always thought that might be a good job for me someday after being a bodyguard. I liked learning how to do that.

I'd also been into acting when I was younger. I had this guy named Maurice De Pena who was a commercial agent. He got me some work around this time. I was always up for anything, so I auditioned for a national Sprite commercial. I landed the part. They ended up casting me just being myself, holding up a big ghetto blaster on my shoulder. The next thing I knew, I was sitting in a trailer, waiting to shoot a Sprite commercial. The only downside to that was that the commercial shot during a trip The Pharcyde made to Japan. I was disappointed I had to sit that one out. But getting to be on TV across the country, even just in a commercial, was a pretty good consolation prize.

12

WAFFLE HOUSE

I was twenty-three when I went on my first outing with The Phar-cyde in the fall of 1992. This was the first time in my life that I'd seen anywhere outside of Los Angeles. It was opening my eyes in all sorts of ways, but not when it came to my weight. Without really even being aware that it was happening, I was getting bigger than ever. I was over 400 pounds then. Of course, I was still agile enough to kick some ass when need be, without getting touched myself, but I was big. And what's a trip is I didn't know how slow and unhealthy I was because I had nothing to compare it to—that's how I'd always felt. I didn't know any better.

For many of us, the things we want to change in our lives but feel powerless over, I think a lot of us become good at looking the other way. It's a big part of how denial works. If we're cool with our faults, because that's just how it is, then we don't have to carry out the hard task of changing. We put off change. We get used to being out of breath, to being uncomfortable, to being broke, to being unhappy at work or at home, whatever it is. Looking back from the other side, it's like I want to say to myself, "Dude, you have no idea how much better it could be to live a healthy lifestyle." But we've all got to crash the car ourselves to get the message. I wasn't there yet.

I knew I was different. It was impossible not to because my life had all sorts of elements that most people never would have known about. Like when I went to the doctor, and they weighed me on one of those moving weight scales, they had to add this hook with an additional 150 pounds because those scales only go up to 350 pounds. So that's how I got my weight. Just like with everything else my weight had affected in my life, I was really good at ignoring it. To this day, I don't know exactly how or why. It could be like I was fat and naïve, or fat and oblivious. What's crazy is that I knew I was big, but somehow, even with the special scale and the number that it went up to when I stood on that platform, I really had no idea how big I was. I didn't see what other people saw when they looked at me.

At the same time, I'd look at people and think, *Damn, that's a big girl.* Not in a judgmental way or anything, but just noticing something out of the ordinary. Like noticing on a 120-degree day, *Damn it's hot.* Even to this day, I'll look at someone and think, *Man, he's big.* And then it will hit me, *I was 150 pounds bigger than that.* But, back then, I couldn't see any of this. I had no perspective at all. In some ways, this was good, because I still had the confidence I'd always had with girls, with rapping, and everything else. And I was mostly pretty happy. I know, even *I* find that somewhat hard to believe, but I've thought about this a lot over the years. It really is the truth. It's not like I think I was supposed to be depressed, or I was supposed to be unhappy. But I didn't see the reality of my weight, or how it impacted my health.

There were moments that made this harder, though. When the group was shooting the video for their song "Runnin,'" I was sitting down during this scene they were filming. The next thing I knew, I was looking at the clouds.

Man, what happened here? I wondered.

I broke the fucking chair. That's what happened. It was embarrassing because people had to help me up and everything. But it didn't fuck up my day.

Even when I was traveling all the time with the band, I wasn't thinking too much about being tight in a seat on an airplane. We were usually rolling through the States on a tour bus anyway, and I always felt comfortable on them.

Being fat actually had its upsides as a bodyguard. A lot of nightclub bouncers are big guys. Some of them would definitely qualify for the morbidly obese range. Once I was doing it for a living, I could see why. Somebody could punch me, hard as they could, right in my gut and it didn't hurt me. I could take anyone slapping me on my arms. That was nothing. My brother Mouse hits like a brick. Same thing, though, when I was big, he could pummel me. It was the one punch I could feel, but it wasn't like he was paralyzing me. The only time I can remember *really* feeling anything was when I was playing around with this fat dude. That man hit me, and I felt the hit. Then it was as if I could feel his fat coming down on me. That's when I was like, *Oh, shit, that's what getting hit feels like.*

Once we started touring a lot, I had eating on the road dialed down. I knew the different restaurants in specific towns we traveled through. At a place where another person would probably get out of the car and take a picture, I'd jump off of the bus and say, "Oh my God, that's a Waffle House."

It did not feel like I was eating all the time, but it was all the time.

The weird thing is, it seemed like during my meals, I'd eat the same amount as someone with a healthy bodyweight. I wasn't eating like my friend Cupid, who's been known to go up to the counter and order four cheeseburgers. I wasn't the guy who'd be like, "Let me get four Big Macs."

My thing was more like, whenever there was food, I'd have some.

"Just let me taste it," I said.

On the road, there was always food.

People who have a healthy bodyweight usually only eat when they're hungry. They wouldn't taste a little of every single item of food they passed by. But with me, there were times, especially early on, when we would get to the venue and the green room backstage was just like a paradise. There'd be chicken. There'd be sandwiches. My guys in the band didn't eat before a show. But I sure did.

"Yeah, I'll have it," I said.

Whatever it was, that was my thing, "I'll have it."

Romye, he loved Hawaiian bread, which are those soft, sweet, round loaves of bread. That was his thing, so there was always some of that around. That was pretty much all any of them ever wanted. The rest of it was for me. I took full advantage. I even planned ahead for future eating. As we were leaving the venue, I'd be getting the bus stocked.

"We need to take some of this on the bus, too," I would say.

I made it seem like that was part of my job, but I knew the band wasn't going to eat the stuff I was grabbing. Really, I was looking out for myself. And so there I was after the show was over, carrying sandwich trays out to the bus. That's how I stayed Big Boy.

13

ON THE ROAD

1993 was pretty much a year on the road. I was so happy. Not only was I getting to see The Pharcyde perform every night, but we were out touring with Tupac Shakur, and all these other cats. It was an amazing experience for me. There were times we'd look out for Pac and make sure he was cool because we had a show together, or because he was a day ahead or a day behind us on the road. This was around the time his song, "I Get Around" was popular, I was a huge fan. Pac was really intelligent. I had a lot of conversations with him on the road that showed me how wise he was. He was a hell of a talker—about music, always, and females. Also, since his parents were in The Black Panthers, he had a lot to say about politics. He was very aware.

But—no disrespect—he could be crazy at the same time. I remember having shows in Ohio canceled because Pac had gone there first and messed something up. When we came along behind him, the promoters didn't want any trouble, so they canceled our show, too. The night that Pac got arrested for beating up his limo driver on the way to a taping of *In Living Color,* we were there; so we all got locked down. That was just how it was with Pac. The other thing was that women loved him. Just being in the same hotel with him, I saw a lot, let me tell you. I can bear witness to how some women would sit outside his door in a line, hoping they would be chosen to come in. At shows, I saw them jump on the stage. I saw them literally tear down a fence trying to get at him once. This could make it wild to get in and out of places.

One time, we did a concert sponsored by the local hip hop station for 30,000 people in Tacoma, Washington. After the show, when it was time to leave the venue for our hotel, Pac jumped in the van with us. Now, with 30,000 people at the show, we got stuck in traffic trying to leave. Our driver was this young Caucasian girl who liked the Pharcyde. She'd been cool to us when she drove us to the show. Well, she must have loved Tupac, because as soon as he got in the van, it was obvious how giddy she was. Pac was in form, clowning and being loud. He was hopping around between the seats in the 15-passenger van we were in. Then, we got into some hard traffic.

Tupac wanted the girl to bounce out of our lane into the lane of oncoming traffic, which was empty, to pass all of the other traffic. I guess Tupac was too much to resist. The next thing we knew, she had whipped into the oncoming traffic lane. We were passing every car that was waiting to get on the highway. The reason everybody was at a standstill was that there was a police officer that had the street blocked off and was mandating how the traffic funneled onto the highway. When he saw this damn van driving the wrong way down the street, he put his hand out and used his flashlight to pull us over. I felt badly because our driver only broke the law because Tupac told her to, but now, she was going to be the one who got in trouble. I tried to help her out. I leaned over and talked to the officer through the driver's side window.

"We got the headliners in the van," I said.

He didn't want to hear that.

"Let me have your license and registration," he said to the girl.

When the girl handed them over, the officer walked over to his car. This whole time, Tupac was being cool.

"We've got time," he said. "We've got time."

The officer wrote the girl a ticket and made us get back into the line of traffic, which was at a standstill. People must have started to figure out that Tupac was in our van because we started to get a few people around us, trying to look in. Just as Tupac pulled out a joint, there was this young girl—she looked about nine years old—outside the window, peering in at him. So he leaned out his window and pulled her close to him.

"What you are about to see me do, I shouldn't have done," he said. "This is very wrong. You can't tell anybody what you seen. This is going to be your secret and my secret—our secret."

Her eyes got so big. She nodded her head yes. To this day, I'm sure she tells that story about her moment with Tupac. And I'm sure the girl who was driving the van that day still tells her story about Tupac. Hell, I'm still telling it. Why? Because he's a legend.

In his twenty-five years, he did so much. But there was more that he could have done and more we could have learned from him. I don't think the masses had a chance to understand what this dude's role could have been. Not to put him on the level of like Martin Luther King Jr. and Malcolm X, but I can't help but think of the similarities. Malcolm X was a former hustler and drug dealer who did his time in prison. He spoke to and for the people. Pac spoke to and for the people. Also, a lot of those leaders died young. A lot of Pac's accolades were posthumous. But even now that he's been gone for a decade, his power hasn't dimmed. When I listen to albums like *Thug Life* or songs like "Dear Mama," it's clear that we had a leader there. I can see it in the way that people hang onto his words, wear their Tupac tattoos with pride, call him preacher, saint, and revolutionary, that he still represents something beyond himself or his music. To me, that's real leadership. Like he said in his own book of poetry, he was *The Rose That Grew from Concrete*. This dude knew what he was talking about. Passing so young, and leaving the legacy that he did, I'm not surprised that people still love him like they do and that people still say that he's their favorite artist. In everything that we have from Pac that was released posthumously, people could still understand the message, which has become all the more powerful since he passed on. I've also heard rappers say that they hid their beef because of Biggie and Tupac; I really think some lives got saved because of that. Given the small time that we did have Pac, his message and his purpose will outlast his so-called days on earth.

* * *

THE PHARCYDE'S "PASSING ME BY" WAS BLOWING up then, and the shows were nuts. People were just going crazy for them. It was great to be a part of all that good energy. We only got into one real serious problem, and it wasn't even group-related. It was race-related.

We had a show in Dayton, Ohio. But we weren't staying in the city. We were a few miles away. The particular area where we were at was woodsy to the point where, when we called room service at the hotel, it went straight to the Denny's restaurant next door. This was small town living.

When we got back to the hotel after the show that night, somebody—probably me—was like, "Man, let's go get something to eat."

So we walked over to Denny's. Not all of the band was there, but I remember there were a couple members, plus crew. All together there were about eight of us.

When we walked in, we weren't expecting any trouble. At the show earlier in the night, the crowd was racially mixed, and it had felt good—the whole show, the vibe, and everything.

Syl and I walked in together and sat down. We noticed that our merchandise guy, Rick, was across the room, and it looked like he was having a problem with this group of white guys. I couldn't hear what he was saying, but I could see him talking with his hands. It looked like something was going down—and not a good something.

"Man, I think Rick's having a problem," I said.

Rick walked away, but as he did, he was looking over his shoulder. He was looking real mad. Finally, he walked over to where we were standing.

"Rick, man, you cool?" I said.

"These motherfuckers over here are talking all this prejudice nigger shit," he said.

"What?" I said, looking over at the guys.

How dare these motherfuckers say that to us? I thought.

Now you've got to think, I'm straight up Los Angeles. We didn't hear that kind of talk where I was from. Now I was just as heated as he was. We had some local dudes with us, and I guess they were kind of used to this kind of thing. Not us. The locals were trying to talk us down, but we weren't hearing it.

As we were standing there as a group, the three white dudes came through with their three ladies, and as they did so, the smallest one looked right at us.

"You all got a problem?" he said.

I put my shoulders up and I tried to make myself look as big and intimidating as I could. I was probably about 400 pounds and some change then, so it wasn't hard. I towered over the guy mouthing off. But he looked me right in the face as he was talking.

"Yeah, well if any of you fucking niggers got a fucking problem with me and my fucking friend, we'll be sitting right the fuck over there," he said.

Not only was he looking up at me, but also, as he said this, he pointed at me. Then, he walked the ladies through us. You know, they very purposefully split us up as a group, and then they went over and sat down in a booth.

Syl was a time bomb. He was ready to explode.

"Syl, calm down," I said. "Hold on for a second, man. Yeah, we got to get 'em, but hold on. They're going to go sit down. And we're going to put a plan together."

Syl wasn't hearing it. He was ready to jump.

"Hold on man," I said. "Let's go back and talk to Suave."

I knew that if we crushed these dudes right there in the restaurant, we'd bring a whole lot of heat on the group. So we got up, went back across the parking lot and into the hotel and knocked on Suave's door.

"Suave, man," we said. "There's some white dudes at this Denny's, man, and they're giving us some nigger shit."

"What!?" he said.

So he gave us the go-ahead, and that was it. I went back to my room, put on my sweats and my steel toe boots. We met back in the lobby. It was me, three other guys from our crew and these locals. When we went back, two of the dudes—the little cat and one big one—were walking up from their cars as we were walking up. Nothing really had to be said because we knew that was them. They knew why we were coming back. I played it cool, but I was thinking: *Dude, these cats went to the car to get knives or a gun because they knew we were coming back.*

I didn't have time to think after that. It all went into fast motion. Syl hit one of their guys with the palm of his hand, and all this blood splattered on the window of the Denny's. The dude fell up against the window. Syl and I were on him. The big dude was what we were worried about, so I figured I'd get in on him. Once he was handled, I turned to that little shit who had mouthed off to me. I snatched him up. He was on his hands and knees on the ground. He didn't know how to really cover himself up. As I was socking him, he was trying to put his shoulder over his ear. And then, I punched him in the head once, and that hurt my hand.

Dude, I'm just going to stomp this motherfucker out, I thought.

So I started kicking him.

This whole time, the girls who were with these guys, and who had walked through us like they were princesses, were inside the Denny's. They were standing at the window, screaming, trying to get out the door. But Suave was holding the door, laughing at them as we were beating the shit out of their men.

We left them dudes on the ground and took off running back to our hotel. Only, there were too many of us running around in the hotel. I didn't want us to draw too much attention to ourselves. So I calmed everyone down and made sure the group got into their rooms first. Then, I got the rest of us inside. As soon as we got upstairs, we started making an escape plan.

"Man, we got to get out of here," Suave said.

So he called our bus driver. I could hear him talking into the phone.

"Hey, man, sorry for waking you up," he said.

Our driver had been asleep because after that show, we had a long drive ahead of us from Ohio to Atlanta. As soon as Suave explained what had happened, however, the guy was up and on his way over to grab us and get us all out of there.

We went up and down the hallway, knocking on everybody's door.

"We got to go," I said. "We got to go."

I got to Fuzzy's door and knocked. He answered, yawning and confused. And, remember, this was when Fuzz was still fresh out of church. He'd never been anywhere.

"Fuzz," I said. "Man, we just destroyed these white boys over at Denny's. We got to get out of here."

"Where are we going?" he asked.

"We're going to Atlanta," I said.

"Do I have time to brush my teeth?" he said.

"You know what, man?" I said. "Brush your teeth and meet us in Atlanta. We're getting the fuck out of here."

He got it then and hurried it up.

Finally, we got everyone rounded up and got the group on the bus. It was chaos. We were tossing our luggage into the undercarriage of the bus. Where we were, it was so woodsy and dark and there was so much racism in the air that it seemed like they could get away with public lynching around there.

As soon as we all climbed onto the bus, the bus driver took off, serious about his mission.

"Turn off all the lights and don't look out the window," he said. "Don't say anything."

So we had our whole bus completely dark. Our driver was Caucasian, and we wanted his face to be the only one visible from the outside. I had my window on the side of the bus cracked and, of course, I couldn't help myself. I peeped out. The town we were in was so small that the sheriff and his wife didn't even have a squad car. They drove around in a burgundy car. A bunch of other cars had pulled up alongside theirs. There were all of these different sheriff cars, no more official looking than theirs, and nothing looked uniform. I don't know if it was other sheriffs or deputies, but they had called a lot of guys in. They all had their lights flashing. We had to drive through all of that to get out of town.

I saw the dudes we had flattened. One of them was still kind of laid out on the ground.

Oh, fuck, I thought.

The girls were talking to the police.

As the bus driver crept through the parking lot, light was flooding through the front of the bus.

Oh shit, oh shit, oh shit. Dude, they're about to stretch us, I thought.

I think the cops were looking for some locals, not the rap group that was staying in town that night. When they saw the tour bus, they waved us through. As we drove away, we looked through the windows. We weren't the avengers we'd been earlier. We were frightened now, our hearts pounding, our hands shaking. After everything we had just seen, we did not want to get stopped in that town.

Finally, we made a turn and drove down the street that led to the interstate. This whole time, we were all silent, looking behind us, waiting to be lit up by a squad car.

As soon as we got on the interstate and started flying along, we became all, "Yeah, yeah, what's up, motherfucker? This is L.A. Fuck you, motherfuckers!"

We knew it could have gone down much differently. Afterwards, we hated to think that a group of local black men might have ended up taking the fall for what we had done, but we couldn't see a way to make sure that didn't happen. All we knew was, with the mood in that town at that moment, we had to get out of there. And I have to say, I would still do the same thing today. Obviously, it would be different because I'm a public figure now. But if faced with the same bigotry, there's no way I would walk out of that restaurant without doing something. Making a stand against that kind of ignorance and hatred is more important than any consequence it might cause.

But, honestly, that was the only problem I ever got into during my years with The Pharcyde. It was a good run.

14

ANOTHER NEAR MISS

By the Spring of 1994, when I was twenty-four, I knew a lot of people in the Los Angeles hip hop scene. I had always been cool with The Baka Boyz, who had a mix show on POWER 106 FM at that time. I had known them when they were doing radio in Bakersfield. They used to come down to Los Angeles to DJ for Paul Stewart. Once they got their show on POWER, they quickly became the top guys at the station. They were like the fathers of the mothership at that time. Their Friday Night Flavas show was humongous. I used to go in sometimes and do a segment with them called "This Be It or Frisbee It," where we'd play a new track and let the listeners decide if "This Be" a hit, or a "Frisbee," as in get it out of here.

Every artist knew them and knew they had to make an appearance there. It was like when I was on the road with The Pharcyde, and there were certain DJs at certain stations we knew we had to visit: In Houston, it was THE BOX on 97.9; in New York City, it was Funk Master Flex on HOT 97; in LA, it was The Baka Boyz on POWER 106. Those dudes were responsible for a lot of people that came through the door in those years. It didn't get any bigger than them.

They deserved the respect, too. When you heard Nick V crack that mic and Eric V on the turntables it was just—it was something magical, a time in hip hop that we haven't had since. The Baka Boyz really worked hard. They carried the station on their backs, creating the station's street team, which is still called the Flavor Unit.

Their popularity was not only a big deal for their show and the station, it was a big deal for hip hop in America. You have to remember that hip hop was still counterculture. It was still on its way up. And POWER was one of the first stations in the country to give it respect and help move it into the mainstream. Before that, people still called it "that ghetto music."

Before POWER and The Baka Boyz, there had been some great records and rappers. There were even some great stations out in L.A. I give props to the original KDAY, which was great and exclusively hip hop. THE BEAT did their thing. KJLH and KACE danced with it. But the reason the K-DAY DJs and The Baka Boyz were so special is that they were mix masters on turntables. We'd tune in, and here were these dudes, cracking these mics, mixing on these turntables, sounding like your neighbor, your homey, the guys in your crew. They weren't polished. They were real.

Back then, The Baka Boyz were known as The Two Fat Mexicans, and I was Big Boy, so I guess we were an obvious unit—like two bacon double cheeseburgers with an extra large side of fries. That Memorial Day weekend, we decided to hit some barbecues. We literally had a sheet of barbecues we were going to drop in at. We were all crammed into their little Ford Festival. I was in the back—well over 400 pounds—while Nick V, at 245 pounds, and Eric, at 225 or 230, stuffed into the front together. Partway through the day, they told me we had to make a detour.

"We've got to stop at our boss's house, man," they said.

"Dude, we're having such a good day," I said. "I really don't want to stop at your boss's house."

"Big, it'll be real quick," they said.

"Alright, fine, let's go," I said.

I was the passenger, so I was going to go wherever they were going. Anyhow, it didn't stop me from clowning.

"Dude, your boss's house?" I said. "Man, this is going to be a white man, his white wife, two white kids, white picket fence."

And as soon as we pulled up, there was this white guy outside, waving at us. And then, it was just like an old TV show: Here was the white wife.

"Hello," she said and waved to us.

And then, their two little white kids bounced over.

Oh shit, I thought, trying not to laugh so hard that they would think I was rude.

And, of course, to get into their yard, I walk through this little white picket fence. So everything I had said—just clowning around—that was exactly what we were walking into.

When we got around to the back of the house, Rick was barbecuing burgers. It wasn't a party or anything. It was just the Cummings family and us. I didn't know who Rick Cummings was. I had no clue that he was the program director for POWER at the time. Or that he was way bigger than putting a title on the door since he had started the company with just one other person. None of that made an impression on me. I wasn't trippin' off what The Baka Boyz did. I'd been in the station with them a few times, but I never thought about doing it myself.

I just happened to be in a good mood that day. So, I was clowning with Rick. I can remember him standing at the grill laughing. I can't remember any of the funny things I said. There was never a moment where I felt like I nailed it or I had been discovered or anything like that. And then, just as quickly as we got there and had our fun, we left. When we were getting in the car, I was actually glad that we had stopped by because it had been a good time.

"Man, your boss is cool," I said. And that was it.

I was still bodyguarding for The Pharcyde. Later that week, we were traveling to San Francisco for a show. I was with the group at their house, getting ready to go catch our flight. Only, this was around the time that OJ Simpson was running from the law. On that particular day, he was in his white Bronco on the freeway with helicopters overhead. The guys were watching this unfold on television. They didn't want to leave and end up missing anything. I was looking at the time, looking at the time, looking at the time—but there was nothing I could do. We missed our flight. We still had to get to the show, so we had to rent a van.

When we went to rent the van, I had a gun on me, a Walther

380 automatic. When I was at home I carried a gun every day, and my gun was always illegal. If I left the house with Fuzz, or whoever, and I forgot my gun, we would have to double back and get it. That was just me. It wasn't like I was going to go rob you or whatever. But I figured if I got into anything, I was going to make the odds even. I called my gun The Equalizer. If someone thought they were going to come at me, I was going to light their ass up and make sure I got home okay.

I always left my gun at home when we flew up and back to San Francisco for a show because I had to go through security at the airport. But I figured I could take it with me since we were driving. We got up there, The Pharcyde did their show and whatever else they had to do. And then, we were hanging out because we were tight with the guys in Hieroglyphics and a few other crews.

"We're going to spend a couple of days up here," Romye said.

"Well I want to go home," I said.

They were cool with that, but I had my gun on me.

"Man, I'm going to fly home," I said. "But I can't fly with my gun."

I tucked it in the van, so it wouldn't get them in trouble if they got stopped.

"When you guys get home, let me know, and I'll come pick up my gun," I said.

And then, I headed to the airport to be on my way.

When I got home and I didn't have my 380, I started carrying another gun, this 25 I had. A few days later, I was driving when the guys in Pharcyde called me.

"Hey, Big, we're home," they said.

"Okay, well, I'm about to come get my gun then."

I was in Culver City at the time. I drove from there over to their house in Los Feliz. We were kicking it. Then, I went home. As soon as I got back into Culver City, the police lit me up. I was in this white Astro van that I had just bought.

A cop came up on the driver's side of the van.

"Get out of the vehicle," he said.

I did. Right away, he searched me. It didn't take long because all I was wearing was shorts, a t-shirt and some corduroy house shoes.

"Sit down," he said.

I sat down on the curb.

"Are there any guns in the vehicle?" he asked.

"No, there's no guns in the vehicle," I said.

He and his partner started searching my van anyway. While they were searching it, they flipped up the carpet and found a stash box. Now, I would never put a stash box right under the driver's seat, where anybody could find it. Just because the person I bought the van from made it—not me—doesn't mean the cops were going to buy that excuse. The cops were certain I had a gun somewhere in the van—or on me—and by this point, they were getting pretty agitated. They kept going through my van, over and over again.

As I sat on the curb watching them, I started to sweat a little bit because I knew I had two warrants out for my arrest. They were nothing crazy, just letting tickets get away from me for moving violations or driving without insurance. But I knew that one day they were going to catch up with me. When they did, I would have to do the days or pay the fine. It was starting to look like this was going to be that day. I was prepared for my day of reckoning. I had told my brother Mouse what to do if I got picked up.

"Man, when they catch up with me on these warrants, don't come bail me out," I told him. "Just let me do the days."

"Okay, cool," he said.

I had saved up a little bit of money, and I didn't want to drop it all on bail.

Finally, the cop came back to where I was sitting on the curb.

"Stand up," he said.

He searched me again: Nothing. He sat me back down.

But he was determined to find something. So he searched my van again.

At this point, I'd been sitting there for about 45 minutes. They had already searched me four times. They ran my name; then he came back over to me.

"Well, you have two outstanding warrants," he said. "We're going to take you in, and we're going to do a detective hold on your van."

I knew that a detective hold meant that they could strip my van and really look for this gun he was so sure that I had because of the stash box. They put me in the squad car, and I watched the tow truck come. They hooked my van up and drove off with it. Then the cops pulled out. They rolled me over to Culver City.

Fuck, I thought.

They got me out of the car and searched me one more time. Then, they put me in this little secured holding area. After they took off my handcuffs, they turned me around and searched me again. That cop had his hands all in my pockets and along my shirt. He was running his fingers along the inseams of my sweat shorts and everywhere. He was real thorough. I guess he thought I sold drugs and had little stashes all over me. But he didn't come up with anything.

Finally, they allowed me my one phone call. I got Mouse on the phone. Mouse and I went through a few rounds of "bail me out."

"Dude, they arrested me on those warrants," I said. "I need you to come and bail me out. I'll pay you back."

"Wait, what's going on man?" he said. "You said don't bail you out."

"Dude, just bail me out," I said.

"Okay," he said, but he still sounded doubtful.

Meanwhile, the cops put me in a cell. I knew that if Mouse didn't bail me out, they were going to process me and take me to the county jail. But there was nothing to do but wait. About thirty minutes later, a guard came in.

"Alexander," he said.

I was looking around at the time, wondering what was going on, *Dude, is it county bus time or they going to move me somewhere else?*

"Someone's here to bail you out," he said.

As I was walking out, I saw Mouse waiting for me. He was looking at me like he was trying to figure out what was going on, but I wouldn't say anything.

"Man, you all right?" he said.

"Yeah," I said. "Thank you."

We walked outside, down the stairs and out onto the street. When we got to his car, I reached under my stomach and pulled out both guns. I weighed so much that I could stash things in my stomach, and I had been able to hide both guns—loaded—under my fat rolls. I knew how to tuck it just right so that, even with everything they made me do—stand up, sit down, everything—the guns never fell out. All those times the cops searched me, they never found them.

But if Mouse hadn't gotten there when he did, I was about to be in some real shit because they were about to take me to the county jail, and once I got there, they would have fully strip searched me. And then, not only would they have found those guns, but also, I would have been in a world of trouble for having them.

By the time Mouse and I got home after all of that, it was around three or four in the morning. I was exhausted, so I lay down and went to sleep. A few hours later, maybe around 10:00 A.M., my phone rang. I didn't recognize the number, but I answered.

"This is Rick Cummings from POWER," he said. "May I speak to Big Boy?"

"Hey, what's going on?"

"I got your number from Nick V."

"Hey, cool."

I had no idea what this call was about. I was waiting to see what he said.

"I want to try something with you," he said. "Have you ever thought about doing radio?"

"No."

"Well, I was wondering if you might want to come in and try one overnight," he said. "We'll give you $35 an hour. Just come in and have some fun on the microphone."

"Alright," I said.

I wasn't thinking about anything more than making a little extra money, but that call launched *Big Boy's Neighborhood*. If I had been in county that day, as I almost was, I would have missed it. A few months later, after I got cool with Rick, I told him, "When you called me I had just gotten home from being arrested."

Like I said, I've had too many near misses not to feel like someone was looking out for me, helping me to get to where I was supposed to be. I simply needed to get out of my own damn way long enough to get there.

15

I CAN'T TEACH YOU TO BE A PERSONALITY

The week that Rick Cummings called me to come in and try out the radio thing, I was home between shows with The Pharcyde. And just like that, with one phone call, I had a new thing to throw against the wall.

I had met Rick on Memorial Day, a Monday. He called me that Wednesday. Later that same week, I went into the POWER 106 studio in Burbank and did my first overnight. That meant going in at midnight and being on the air until 5:30 A.M. Then The Baka Boyz came on and did the morning show. Even though I had never thought about doing radio before, and I didn't have any idea what I was doing, Rick made it easy for me. When I first came into the studio, Rick sat me down and laid it all out for me.

"I hear something in you," he said. "I can teach you radio, but I can't teach you to be a personality. You have personality, so I can teach you radio."

That made sense to me. I was used to being known for my big personality as much as for my big size. I waited to see if he had any other advice for me.

"Go in there and have fun," he said. "Be yourself. Do what you want to do. Just remember that the station is called POWER 106."

"Alright," I said.

From there, I walked into the studio, met my engineer and got set up. In my mind, all I was thinking about was having fun, introducing the songs, maybe popping a couple listener calls on the air, and remembering that I was at POWER 106.

So I started doing my show, and what did I go and say?

"This is Big Boy on POWER 107."

Power 107, where did that come from?

The next morning, Rick listened to the tape. Besides my one little slip up, he must have heard something. He called me at the house later that day.

"I heard your tape," he said. "Would you like to try it again?"

In my mind, I wasn't tripping about a radio career. I was just doing the math: that was two days of work at $35 per hour, and that sounded good to me.

I really didn't think about it too much more than that. I didn't know any better. Today, there are cats who are trying to get into radio, and they hear how to act on the air by listening to Big Boy, Mickey Fickey Mix, Eric D-Lux, and they think that's the way it's done: You've got to make noise. You've got to clown. You've got to have bits.

I came up the ranks when it was much more straightforward. DJs introduced the songs in a more direct way. It was more about the station's brand than the personality of any one DJ. I came into that, but that wasn't me. If I had gone to school and studied radio, or if I had always wanted to be a radio guy, I probably would have followed that same pattern. And who knows if I would have had the career that I've had. Instead, I was just being myself. To the listeners, I sounded like their neighbor, their partner, somebody they went to school with, their crew. I was familiar. It was not hard for people in L.A. to identify with this big black guy that had never done radio and sounded pretty much just like them.

I did go in with a few ideas because I was like, *Man, what am I going to talk about?* So I had this little tablet of paper, and I wrote down everything I could think of that might be funny to do on the air. One idea was to do a "Whisper In." Everybody was all about "Shout Outs" back then, so I thought the thing to do was to have a whisper in, where I talked real quiet and gentle like I had a headache. It was a cool idea, and listeners liked it, but it burnt out quick. I soon learned that's how it was with some bits—they had a bigger impact in my mind than they did on the air.

Other than that, I was just being myself, Big Boy.

After two overnights, Rick called me at my house again and asked me if I wanted to do the night show permanently, which was from 7:00 P.M. to midnight.

"Yeah, I guess," I said.

I was totally taken by surprise. To be honest, I didn't really listen to the station that much. I didn't know they were hiring at the moment. I still wasn't even sure how I'd gotten the gig. I think Rick just saw good energy and the fact that I was a big, happy guy. Now he had the Two Fat Mexicans, and he had Big Boy. Once I started, I think that personality came into play because I was good with joking with listeners and guests, turning a joke on myself, or just having fun. Around that same time, Coolio asked me to do the video for his song "Fantastic Voyage." I had known him for a few years through Paul Stewart. The video aired right around the same time I started at POWER, so that was like a calling card for me. If people didn't know who I was, I could point to this video that was everywhere.

While I was starting up at POWER, I tried to hold onto everything else. I was still The Pharcyde's bodyguard, and I figured I could do both jobs. I didn't know how serious a radio career was, so in the beginning, I would work during the week at POWER 106 and then go out with The Pharcyde on the weekend. This was the spring or summer of 1994. They were playing Lollapalooza on the weekends.

But I don't think I lasted even three weeks. That first weekend, The Pharcyde's show was in the Bay Area. And even though that required almost no traveling at all, I realized what a grind it was. So I had a talk with myself. At first I decided that I was not going to do this radio thing. I was going to stay out on the road with The Pharcyde because I loved being out there. I loved seeing the group perform. And I loved getting to perform with them when I filled in for Fat Lip. This didn't happen enough for me to think that I was going to make it my main gig, but I still dreamed about being a rapper. When I was on the side of the stage, looking out for the guys, I'd get this thing where I wished that the crowd was out there for me. I was smart enough to know that this wasn't the best place for a bodyguard to be at, since my attention needed to be fully focused on my own job to keep everybody safe. But I'd wanted to rap for too long not to get those kinds of urges.

I was reasonable about where I was at though, and I figured that even if I didn't make it as a rapper, if my time as a bodyguard was coming to an end, I really liked being on the road. I figured that maybe I could become a tour manager or a manager.

Around then, this other group called Another Level was starting to get a little recognition. I had done some bodyguarding for them when I was on break from The Pharcyde, and then I got into kind of road managing them.

So I figured that was it, I was going to quit radio and be a road manager. At the same time, if someone had come up to me and offered me a deal to release a rap record for Def Jam, I would have taken that, too.

And then, during my final weekend with The Pharcyde, I had a conversation with Fuzzy where we were kicking around the idea that, as a bodyguard or road manager, I could only eat when The Pharcyde ate. My success was really based on their success. When they stopped, I stopped. Around this time, things were starting to slow down because they were between albums, which meant they were home more. I didn't want to keep leapfrogging from gig to gig and group to group. So I decided that maybe I needed to try to do something for myself. I would take the radio thing more seriously.

There are some people that are locked in on a certain thing they want to do. Not me. I was all over the place. And that's why I say this life that I have now was just willed to me. I mean, imagine if I had quit POWER like I planned and stayed out on the road. But with the big decisions that I've made in my life, it's been more like—let me just back up, let go and let God. When I've done that, it has all worked out.

I sat down with The Pharcyde and told them my decision. They gave me their blessing, and my focus shifted to radio. I figured I would just try it. If it didn't work out, that was cool. But once I started, I never looked back. Out of everything I had happened to throw up against the wall—phone scams, rapping, DJ'ing, bodyguarding—radio just happened to stick.

Once I was committed to my gig on POWER, I got into some of the bits that people still identify me with. When I first started, the overnight timeslot was Big Boy and Richard Humpty Vission at night; so we were both doing different things, adding our own humor to the show. Humpty always led the talk breaks. Probably the first thing I did was "The Dreidel Song," which I had learned when I took Hebrew in fourth grade. I don't know how it even came to me, but one night, Humpty put on this *Lords of the Underground* instrumental track. He was talking, and I just started singing "The Dreidel Song," in Hebrew, over the instrumental. I didn't think it was going to blow up at all. But people went crazy for that. I'd be out after that and black cats, white cats, Mexican cats, they'd all be like, "Man, sing that 'Dreidel Song'."

People still come up to me and ask me to sing "The Dreidel Song." The same thing happened with what became one of my biggest trademarks—"Shaking My Ass." That was another one that I had no idea would take off. It was just another case of Humpty playing the instrumental track in the studio, and while he was talking over it, I was like: "Man, this song right here, just listening to it makes me feel like shaking my ass." So I just started clowning and freestyling and before I knew it, I had come up with this song, "Shaking My Ass." After that, every night, I would do "Shaking My Ass," and people started calling in to request it. My friend Geo told me this story once about how he was at a club in L.A. passing out promotional materials. He approached this group of women and started chatting them up.

"Are you coming in ladies?" he said.

"Yeah, we're going to come in after Big Boy does 'Shaking My Ass,'" they said.

"Oh, okay," he said.

He walked away thinking, *Woah, Big Boy's shit is blowing up!*

Humpty and I always had regular meetings with the station managers. They would give us the pros and cons of what we had done the night before. Pretty soon, it seemed like all the good stuff was Big Boy and all the other stuff was Humpty. One day, Humpty was shaking his head as we left a meeting.

"Hey, bro, they're going to want you to do this by yourself," he said.

"No, man, we're a team."

"No, bro, they're going to want you to do this yourself."

Not long after that, one of the station managers called me into his office.

"Hey, tonight, go in there by yourself," he said.

This was the big time.

Oh shit, this is it, I thought.

So I went in that night, and I sucked. I don't know why. It just totally fell flat without Humpty there, and I knew it.

The next morning, Rick Cummings called me.

"Yeah, it wasn't what I thought it was going to be," he said. "Maybe you do need Humpty in there."

When I heard him say that, I immediately felt determined to prove him wrong.

"Let me try it one more time," I said.

I still don't know exactly what it was that Rick saw in me, but he let me try again on my own. And I went in there and blew it out of the water. I guess I had figured out my game. Ever since then, I've been solo with a crew backing me up.

16

RAP ATTACK

This whole time, when I first started working at POWER, I had a board operator named Flounder. He was like my security blanket. I was supposed to get in there and learn the board, which is how we cued up the CDs and played the promos between songs and answered calls. But even though I had DJ'd for years, since I had no real radio experience, it was a whole different game. I was nervous about running the board on my own, since I had Flounder do it for me for about three months. I also had a girl named Donna who answered the phones. They happily became a part of the craziness of the night show.

But a few months in, Rick sat Flounder down.

"Big Boy running the board yet?" Rick asked.

"No," Flounder said.

"He's not?" Rick said. "Well, he has to run his board tonight."

"I don't think he can," Flounder said.

"Well, let him run Rap Attack," Rick said.

Speaking of attacks, I almost had a heart attack when Flounder told me this. Rap Attack was the hardest part of the show to run. Today, we've got computers. DJs can edit the mix together in advance. Not back then. Rap Attack was like a rap battle between two songs. The songs were on CD, so I had to put both CDs in the

CD player. And then, I had to have an instrumental cart for the music that played in between them. I'd get all of that lined up. Then, I'd get on the mic.

"Rap Attack, here's the champion," I said. "Fu-Schnickens 'Break Down.'"

I would hit the play button and let that song play. Once the song was over, I fired that instrumental cart. And then I did my next bit on the mic.

"Yeah, POWER 106, *Big Boy's Neighborhood,* we've got Rap Attack going on. That was the champion right there. Now we're about to go into the challenger."

Then, I had to hit another button to do the musical bit. And then, play the CD. While that was playing, I had to cue up the instrumental cart again and then take this other cart and go back to the beginning so that after the CD was over, the first instrumental bit played again. At the end, I hit the mic again.

"That was the challenger right there. Call us up. Call us up. And vote for Rap Attack."

I had to man the phone lines while keeping the whole thing going, too.

"POWER 106, *Big Boy's Neighborhood,* you guys are voting. This is what you're voting on. Here's the champion."

Hit that song.

"Here's the challenger."

Hit that song.

And it went on and on, just playing bits of the Rap Attack champion and the Rap Attack challenger, until the voting was done. Managing all of that was pretty much the hardest thing possible. Rick just threw me right in there to learn it.

With the way I sweated doing my first night of Rap Attack, I knew that I needed a little more practice on the board. Even though I was now regularly running the board during Rap Attack, I also took to scheduling in some overnights, where it wasn't as crucial if I made a mistake. So I went in there, ran the board during the overnights a little bit, until I started feeling more comfortable. But we had like five or six hours of overnight to fill. And so we had to figure out how to pass the time. So, out of boredom, Flounder would call somebody. And we recorded it just on the reel-to-reel tape, not live on-air. I would get the person on the phone, "Hey, wonder if you could come by."

I think one of the first ones we did was calling the 24-hour grocery store, Vons, which was down the street from the station. When we got them on the line, we just clowned them a little. But we were rolling, and it passed the time. We recorded all of this onto reel-to-reel. We never did anything with it. But I always had them in my locker.

One of the craziest parts of being on the radio was that suddenly I was interviewing cats that I'd known forever. I remember when I first got to the station, The Pharcyde's first album was already being played, and so I was happy to give it even more love and bring them into the studio with me. The first time they came in for an interview, they could not get over how much things had changed.

Imani just kept looking at me and shaking his head.

"Dude, this is crazy," he said. "Dude, you're asking us questions. Dude, this is crazy."

I also had the chance to interview Run D.M.C., which was a big deal for me. They were sitting in the studio with me. I was flashing back to seeing them play at standing room only concerts in the early days. And now, even though I wasn't rapping like I'd thought I'd be, we were in the music business together. Since I had been a fan, when those cats came in, I already had a vested interest in them and their music. Helping to spread the word felt amazing. Another huge interview for me was Ice Cube—not only because I was such a big fan. He had this song called "Grand Finale" with the opening line "Picture a N-word that's raw," that had this line in it that had always troubled me, "Fuck the father." I had thought it meant "Fuck God." When Ice Cube came into the studio, after I asked him a few questions, I got right down to it.

"What's that line mean?" I asked.

"Fuck my daddy," he said.

That was one thing that I could never get an answer to until I got to POWER. Now I knew. I loved being on the inside like that.

Not that all of the interviews went that well. One of the first ones I ever did was also one of the worst interviews I've done to this day.

It was with Bone Thugs-n-Harmony. They just started flipping me attitude from second one.

"How long you been together?" I asked.

"Forever," they said.

"How old are you?" I said.

"Old enough," they said.

Now I didn't get this at all because we were both new to our career. They were green as a group, having just gotten their major deal. I was just coming up as a DJ, too. But we were cut from different cloth. When I got my break, I was so grateful. I brought my cats in on it with me. I had my old crew Shaun Juan and DJ Ray working in the station with me because I was in it with those guys. I mean, Ray used to drive me to work. He used to drive my Mom to work sometimes because she still didn't have a car. That's some friendship right there. So when I tangled with Bone Thugs-n-Harmony and got where they were coming from, which was all about being these young punks with attitude, I just wasn't having it.

I didn't even finish the interview. I turned the mics off right there and stopped. It wasn't like I threw them out of the station. We talked until we reached an understanding and there weren't any hard feelings when they left. But, in the moment, I was pissed. Of course, they've been on the show so many times since then, and it's always been great. We all laugh about it now. But they know that they're still the worst interview I've ever done.

Another one I had a problem with was Timbaland. I had Missy on the show, and Timbaland was sitting in the studio while I was talking to her, just reading the newspaper. Since he was there, I threw a little love at him.

"Hey, Timbaland, what's going on with you music-wise?" I said.

"Oh, nothing," he said.

I was not about to be disrespected on my show, so I turned off the mic.

"Ya'll gotta go," I said.

My producer, Jason, could see I was pissed and he backed me.

"Tell them to leave," he said.

So that was it. They were out. Timbaland tried to get me on the phone the whole rest of the day. The thing is, I don't have a panic switch where I'm so upset that I want you to call me so we can go to dinner and talk it out. I don't need an apology. I don't need Timbaland. And Timbaland don't need me. But his people kept calling and calling. Finally, I got on the phone with him. He thanked me for calling him on his attitude. We're cool now. But that moment was definitely not cool.

Happenings like that have been rare, though. Mostly, I have always felt blessed when it came to my new job and life.

17

I'M RICH

When I first started at POWER, the station told me that they wanted to put me under contract. I didn't know anything about that kind of thing, so I went to lunch with my old crew, The Baka Boyz, to get the inside skinny.

"They want to put me under contract," I said. "How much should I ask for?"

Nick took his phone, typed something in and then showed it to me.

I leaned forward and looked at his phone. It said, $35,000.

"Man, I can't ask for no $35,000," I said. "If I ask for $35,000, they're going to not hire me. I'm going to fuck this job up."

"Nah, I think you can get it," Nick said.

"Dude, I'm not going in there asking for $35,000," I said.

"Just see if you can get it," he said.

I nodded my head. But, in my mind, I was like, *Hell no.*

A few days later, I went to a meeting at the station. They gave me a one-sheet deal with all of my contract details on it. They slid it to me across the table, face down, so I had to turn it over to read it. For salary, it said $50,000.

$50,000! I thought.

As soon as I walked out, I called my Mom.

"Mom, I'm making $50,000 a year," I said.

And I called my boy Fuzz.

"Fuzz, $50,000," I said. "Man, how do you spend $50,000 a year?"

I was twenty-four years old. Suddenly, I was making $50,000 a year. And I was ready to make a few changes in my life. When I got home that night, Mom and I celebrated my good news. Only I had to break some bad news to her, too.

"Mom, I'm going to go get an apartment," I said.

She started to cry. Everybody was her baby, even me.

"Your friends are going to be over at your house all the time," she said.

"Mom, I got to go," I said.

I knew that she worried that I was too kind-hearted and that my house would be the hang out . She didn't want people to take advantage of me. I don't know why, our house wasn't a gathering spot for my friends when I was living with her. I think she just wanted me to stay with her.

I found a two-bedroom apartment in Burbank that was about three minutes from the station. When I moved in, I literally didn't have anything because I'd lived with Mom my whole life. I had to buy everything. But that was cool with me. You couldn't tell me I wasn't rich. I mean I was *rich*. I went into this furniture store, and the guy was on the phone. My whole aura was, *How dare you be on the phone? What are you doing? I'm rich.*

Finally, my man got off the phone. He came over to where I was looking at the furniture that I wanted for my apartment.

"May I help you?" he asked.

I was standing in the corner, and I pointed at the living room display.

"I want this," I said.

"What?" he said.

"Just what I'm looking at in this corner right here," I said. "All of that."

In the corner was a black sofa and loveseat with these bronze metallic stripes on the fabric, a coffee table that was a black panther in a crawling position with a sheet of glass on his back and one of those lamps with the multi-bulbs that hung down from the ceiling. I purchased it all. I actually spent so much money that the guy gave me the matching panther book ends with fake diamond eyes.

So I had a two-bedroom apartment, and that was crazy. For one, I had never had my own bedroom in my whole life. To have an extra bedroom, man, that was like bliss. I didn't even know what to do with all that space. I figured I'd make an office for myself. As far as I was concerned, I had enough space for The Lakers to practice in. I bought one of those bedroom sets you see advertised when you're driving down the street—five pieces for $399—and I got a 32-inch TV for my living room. I would literally turn off the TV, walk into my bedroom and then come back into the living room, just to look at that TV.

From there, I ended up moving to the outskirts of North Hollywood and renting a three-bedroom house that had a swimming pool in the backyard. Now I had *two* extra bedrooms. You would have thought I was going to be on the next episode of MTV *Cribs*. In my bedroom, I had a king-sized bed. This room was so small that the door scraped the footboard when I closed it. The only way I could fit the nightstand into the room was to put it at the footboard and then push it forward between the bed and the wall. Even then, it just barely fit. The house had no central air or heating, so I put an air conditioner in the window. Then I had a TV room that was just a sofa and the big TV. The other room was an office. You couldn't tell me nothing bad about that house. I was a king!

I had come a long way from the days when I carried all of my belongings in plastic bags from motel to motel. I was determined that my family was going to come with me. I didn't know how long this radio thing was going to last, so as soon as I could put together enough money, which took about six months of saving absolutely everything, I bought a house for my Mom. I was still renting my place, but my priority was to take care of her first. Out of everything I've accomplished, this is the thing that I'm most proud of. After how hard she worked, and how much she struggled for us seven kids—and after all of the times when we didn't have a place of our own, and knowing how much that must have hurt her—finally, I wanted our family to have a home. I never wanted any landlord or motel manager to ever again have the power to come in and tell her that we had to pack up everything and leave. I never wanted my brothers and sisters or my nephews and nieces to experience that, either. So I made sure we were all good.

Telling her the good news was amazing. It was around Christmas when I went over to the place that she was renting in Culver City. It was the same three-bedroom house I'd been living at until I started at POWER and got my own place, and my brother Keith and my sisters Sheila, Sherrille, and Nicole still lived with her. Charlene had ended up moving home to help our mom out financially, too.

Mom fussed over me for as long as I would let her and fixed me something to eat. When I sat down with her in the cramped living room, I looked around at her possessions and thought about all that we had lost over the years. She had so little to show for her hard work because of everything she had done for us kids. Finally, I was going to be able to do something for her.

"What do you want for Christmas, Mom?" I asked.

"I don't need anything," she said, smiling at me.

"Mom, I want to buy you a house for Christmas," I said.

"No, baby, save your money," she said. "Don't."

"No, Mom, go pick out a house," I said.

When she got that it was really happening, she gave me the biggest hug and one of her big wet kisses. And then she just sat there, crying and crying.

She found a place that she liked in Culver City. We both went and walked through the rooms together.

"You will never have to leave this house," I told her.

That was real important to me. She'd never had her name, Ida Alexander, on a deed before. We were always on a lease for somebody else's place. So I wanted her, and the family, to finally have something that was just for us. My proudest moment was handing Mom the keys to that house and saying, "This is yours."

Of course, I'd never purchased a house. No one in my family had ever purchased a house. I knew what the down payment was, but beyond that, I didn't know what I was doing. I was just signing. And then, after everything went through, I had closing costs of $16,444.

I didn't know what closing costs were, so I hadn't planned for that extra money. With the down payment, and with the closings costs, it totally killed me. I was so broke that I couldn't pay my own rent. I had to come to the station and take an advance against my next few paychecks. But I didn't care. All I cared about was that I'd gotten that house out of the way and taken care of Mom. To this day, I own that house. There's no payments on it or anything. So even if it's a worst-case scenario, and everybody in my family has to live together, we've got a place. After how I grew up, I'll probably think in terms of worst-case scenarios for the rest of my life.

THINGS WERE GOOD IN MY LIFE AND with my family. But my old ways weren't completely behind me. One night after I'd started working at POWER, I stopped at a donut shop. I was in there, talking to the overnight guy, and I watched through the window as the police drove by and looked in at us. They threw a U-turn and came back by again. Then they threw another U-turn and passed by a third time. There was nothing to do but go out and get in my car and head home. When I got into the car, it was like all I had to do was just come out of the donut shop parking lot and literally drive through one green light, and BOOM, they lit me up.

As soon as they pulled me over, they got me out of the car and searched me. The cop turned his attention to my car.

"Can I search your car?" he asked.

I nodded, not really thinking about what was in there. Although I usually carried my gun with me, I hadn't grabbed it before I left the house because the donut shop was so close to where I lived.

Then, as I watched him reach into the console between the seats, I saw was his whole body tense up. I knew what he'd found.

Oh shit, I thought. I must have forgotten to bring it into the house when I got home earlier in the night. If I'd known it was there, I would have tucked it in my stomach, like I'd done when I got arrested before.

"Gun!" he yelled.

I knew I was in for it then. When they went into my wallet, I had stripped gas cards, and not because I needed them either. I was working at POWER, and I was blessed. It was just an old bad habit.

When I got to jail, the same cop searched me again, but more thoroughly this time.

"Pick up your stomach," he said.

Damn, I thought, doing as I'd been told.

Of course, there was nothing for him to find this time since they already had the gun from my car, but it made me feel even luckier about how I'd gotten away with stashing my guns in my stomach the other time. At some point, the cops must have gotten hip to the fact that fat boys had a special hiding place because I've even seen it as a plotline on a cop TV show.

So, I got arrested for carrying a concealed weapon and caught a gun possession case while I was working at POWER. To this day, every time I go through immigration when I travel, I've got to bring a letter from my lawyer. But I brought it on myself. And the good thing was that it made me wiser, right then and there, at age twenty-five or twenty-six. After that, I did not ever again mess around with anything that might have cost me my blessings.

18

A CHANGING OF THE GUARD

I had hit my stride after a year and a half of nights at POWER, and I was number one in my time slot. No one else at that time could touch me. That gave me a little traction at the station. Soon after that, they moved me to Drive Time in the afternoons, which was a higher profile spot. The ratings for the show they had in that slot started dropping. They had this cat, Dave Morales, holding the spot until they found someone who could turn it around. They decided to put me in there weekdays from 3:00 P.M. to 7:00 P.M.

What they wanted was for me to take down this guy named Theo at THE BEAT who was killing it in the ratings. So they put me in to see if I could get at him. I called Theo the L.A. Beast. He was this sexy, athletic Asian guy with a deep voice who was suave and just a master at popping people on the phone. What I mean by that is when he would come out of a song, he'd be in conversation with an artist, and listeners just ate that up.

The competition at that time was between POWER and THE BEAT, period. And it was fierce. KROQ was on its own island, and KISS was a totally different thing, because neither of them played hip hop. They weren't strong competition for us. It was POWER and THE BEAT; and it was a constant struggle. One show on POWER would beat the show at the same time slot on THE BEAT. Then a show at another time slot on THE BEAT would kill its competitor on POWER. There was not one clear winner between the two. And hip hop artists were in a tug-of-war, like which show should they do? *Power House* on POWER or *Summer Jam* on THE BEAT? By then, hip hop had gone from being counterculture to being all about radio. Doing the right show could blow someone up and guarantee a crowd at their L.A. appearance. It was as big of a deal for the artists as it was for the DJs.

Even though ratings are everything in radio, I've never been a numbers guy. For me, it was just one of those things where I knew Theo was there, but it wasn't like my whole outlook was that I needed to beat him. If I did a good show, if I made today better than yesterday, if then I made tomorrow better than today, I knew I'd come out on top.

At first during Drive Time, we were hitting old school a little bit more. At 4:00 P.M., we did this thing called The Funky Four Plus One More, where we played four old school songs, and then one more. But then the old school wasn't testing as well anymore with listeners, so we changed it to Count Down at 4:00, which were the top four songs at the time. People would call in and announce the number three and number two songs, and then we would give them a prize. I called this segment *Big Boy's Neighborhood*. Truth be told, I got the idea from that children's show, *Mr. Roger's Neighborhood*. Inspiration comes from all over, you know? With the way I was living at the time, I'm just surprised I didn't get my inspiration from a show on the Food Network.

Anyhow, other than that one new addition, my afternoon show was basically what I'd always been known for: hot songs, sure, but mostly crazy antics and stuff that people weren't used to hearing because other radio hosts weren't doing it. At the time it was me, DJ Ray and Shaun Juan, with a few noisemakers, a few guests. And then at 4 P.M., when we did the countdown, that was *Big Boy's Neighborhood*: "It's time to get into Big Boy's Neighborhood!"

Working afternoons was a whole different thing. When I had worked nights, none of the sales staff was there at the station that late. So it was just me and my board operator Flounder and our phone operator Donna. We were this tight family, and we had the run of the place.

The only time I was ever in the hallways at the station during the day was when I had to go in for meetings. I didn't know anyone, especially at first. When I started on afternoons, there was so much movement in the hallways—sales people walking by and looking in the window of the studio—it was really weird for me. I had never had to perform like that. So they had to put up blinds in the studio and ask people not to come into the studio while we were on the air, just so I could have that feeling that we were still there all alone. That was the best way for me to create and do the job that I had to do.

The differences at the station during the day took some getting used to, but the schedule was great. The only downside was that if I was out anywhere, I had to break up my day to go into the studio. I could stay out until 2:00 or 3:00 A.M., then sleep late, say until noon, stay at the house until 2:00 P.M., then it was time to go into the station. And I got off early enough that I could still go to the movies. Or I could go do a club at night.

By this time, Big Boy was enough of a name that I was getting paid to do a lot of appearances at clubs around the city, just stopping by to blow up an event. This was around 1998 and 1999; so the clubs that were the hot spots at the time were Daily Planet and Florentine Gardens in Hollywood, Caddies in Alhambra, and Peppers, which was located in the City of Industry. Peppers was like my home plate. I'd be on the air during the day, talking about how I was going to be hitting it that night. And then, when I got there, so many listeners always turned out that it was thunderous. No matter where I was, it was all fun. You couldn't tell me I wasn't living the life. I was in paradise.

It seemed like my profile kept rising. With that came all sorts of things. During those years, I was in a seven-year relationship. I never stepped out on my girl, but I definitely noticed an increase in the ladies gravitating towards me. They knew exactly who I was now. I got chased after more than I ever had before.

I started to feel like I was an ambassador for hip hop. That was such a privilege. I was still coming at hip hop as a fan first. I've never been one to play the Big Boy card; so even at important moments, or when I've had the most momentum, I never realized how popular I was. But, suddenly, I had rappers come into the station and tell me that they felt like their record had popped because they'd been on the show with Big Boy. Or, out-of-town groups were telling me that they'd been schooled by local cats: "I heard when I came to L.A. I had to do your show." It felt like I was right there in the thick of it, like when a record had to be presented, it had to be presented by Big Boy. When somebody had to be validated, they had to be validated by Big Boy and POWER 106. It was crazy! Artists that I had looked up to since I'd gotten into radio, or even since I was a kid, valued my opinion and wanted to hang out. They pulled me into their world by telling me they were shooting a video and wanted me to come by.

I got called, along with a lot of different people, to do a cameo in one of the last Eazy-E videos. I was like, *Damn.* It didn't stop there, either. I've always been a big fan of Wyclef Jean and his song, "Gone Till November." When he did the remix, he called and said, "Big, I got a part for you. Come do this."

Probably one of my biggest thrills came when Ice Cube hit me up to be in his movie, *The Players Club,* which came out in 1998. Cube is a businessman first; so even though he was down with *Big Boy's Neighborhood,* he had me audition. I auditioned, and he gave me the part. That was the biggest thing for me at that time: *I'm doing a movie with Cube. I'm on a movie set with a guy that I pay money out of my pocket to go see in concert.* I learned so much from that time with Cube, just like I did when I was The Pharcyde's bodyguard. I saw how he had built such an empire through his hard work. How he took his business very seriously. How he stayed scandal free, and how he and his queen Kim went home together at the end of the day.

During that shoot, I saw that he wasn't just Ice Cube, the rapper, he was also Ice Cube, the director and actor. I saw how he balanced Lynch Mob and his crew with the fact that this was his work. John Singleton, who had given him his start with *Boyz n the Hood* was on the set. It was an amazing experience, seeing John give Ice Cube pointers. And at the end of it, I was really trippin' because I was like, *I'm walking the red carpet at the premiere of Cube's new movie.*

For a while there, I was on the scene. You could open up a can of Pepsi, and if I knew you was going to open it, and you wanted me there, I'd be like, "Hey man, I'm over here at this Pepsi can opening ceremony that's going on."

But then, it got to the point where I was just like, *Let me do the radio and leave it at that.* I was cool with being Big Boy when it came to POWER 106. For everything else, I felt more comfortable being more in the background. Even with the videos, after awhile, I just kind of stopped doing them because it really wasn't me. I'm not a video whore. If I go to a video shoot now, it's just for support. That's enough. And I don't run out to be at everything as much.

After over a year in the Drive Time slot, I finally started getting the artists over to my show instead of Theo's show. And eventually, people in the city turned us on more during that time of day. That finally put a crack in Theo's numbers. From there, it took us another six months, but we finally beat Theo. And we didn't just beat him. We beat him across the board, in all listener demographics. Like I said, I was never the ratings guy. But here I was, just having fun doing what I was doing, and the ratings followed. That was a good feeling.

Of course, right when we started celebrating, things changed once again. I was soon summoned by the powers that be and asked if I could meet with them later that day. When I went into the office for a meeting with our general manager, Marie Kordus, and our program director, Michelle Mercer, I sat back and waited to hear what they had to say.

"We're thinking about making a switch, and we'd like for you to do mornings."

I knew that the morning numbers were very bad at that time. I didn't want to take that on. It was The Baka Boyz's show. They were the ones who had landed me my gig in the first place. Not to mention that I sometimes got up to go piss at 7:30am., and when I looked at the clock and saw how early it was, I always laughed and said, "Dude, The Baka Boyz are at work right now." And then, I went back to bed. That was how I liked it. That time of the morning seemed too early to me. I was like, *I'm in radio, man, not on the chain gang.*

I sat and thought about it for a minute, though I already knew my answer.

"Man, I'm not doing mornings," I said.

"Well, you know, it's not for sure yet," they said. "Just think about it. But you can't tell The Baka Boyz."

"The Baka Boyz are my friends," I said. "I can't promise I won't tell them. If there's something going on with them, I can't look at them and not say anything."

"Well, we'd rather you not."

"I can't do that," I said.

So I turned down the offer and figured that was that.

As I was walking out of the office, I ran into Eric V. My heart sank when I saw him and thought about the meeting I'd just had. I knew I had to come clean.

"Eric, I need to holler at you," I said.

"What's up?" he said.

"Eric, man," I said. "They just brought me in and they talked to me about doing mornings."

"It's cool, Big," he said.

I knew I'd been asked not to say anything, but it was just something I felt I had to do.

And then, Eric pulled his hat off and started pointing at the gray hair on the side of his head, showing me how stressful the mornings were.

"Okay, cool, cool," I said, laughing.

And that's exactly how I felt—I was cool with where I was at. I could still do everything I wanted to do socially. I didn't have to work weekends. And at that time, a four-hour shift really meant a four-hour shift. There wasn't a lot of prep work before the show. I didn't have to do too much afterwards, either. It was in and out. It was a good life.

I continued to be happy with where I was at. No one at the station brought up me doing mornings again, so I kind of let it go. And then, a few months later, the ratings came out again. The Baka Boyz were even lower than they'd been before. I was still number one in afternoons. The station managers called me in for another meeting.

"We've got to make that flip," they said.

I was still resistant. They kept offering me more and more money, but it didn't matter.

"I don't want to do it," I said.

But, finally, they weren't really asking me. They talked with The Baka Boyz about it. They gave me a raise. They let us all know, "This is going to be what it is."

So I took over the mornings in 1997. The Baka Boyz moved to

cover my spot at Drive Time. After being in there at mornings for a week, maybe two weeks at the most, I was not feeling it.

The mornings were all about ratings. Plus, it wasn't like I was handed good numbers and could build on top of that. Nights had never been horrible at POWER, so I had started out in a good spot without even realizing it at the time. Plus, once I saw what my raise looked like after taxes, that perk was busted. So I went back into that office. I laid it down.

"Put me back in my time slot," I said. "I don't want to do this."

AT POWER BACK THEN, THERE WERE CERTAIN time slots where all the DJ had to do was play music and it was all good. Whatever he brought to the table just added to the show. Mornings were not like that. Suddenly, I was morning, and that meant I was the franchise. There was a lot of pressure to do well. I was up against John London at THE BEAT. He was another one who was just a beast. It wasn't that I was worried about the competition. Even with the added pressure, I still wasn't a numbers guy. Still, I had to take the whole thing a lot more seriously. I realized that everything I had been doing—the cute little songs, the gags and other bits—they were not going to cut it. It wasn't enough to just go buck wild and have fun. I still had to be entertaining, but I also had to have some substance. I had to become news now. I had to become knowledgeable. That was a different monster.

And to make it more challenging, it was harder to get guests on in the morning. At night and in the afternoons, it had been easy because they were already out on the move at that time. But a lot of them were like, "Ah, I'm not a morning person." Usually, they would still come and do the show, but it was harder. And that was the exact moment when we were really trying to get even more A-list artists, as opposed to bringing anyone in. It wasn't enough to have the star's dog trainer in now. We needed the star.

Up until that moment, The Baka Boyz had pretty much run the station. Coming into their time slot behind them was intense. But I dug in. Over time, I made it work. The pressure to come up with new, stronger material also meant that I ended up introducing a running bit that has become one of my signatures. When I got moved to the morning show, I worked with two different producers. Then I hired Jason Ryan. Together, he and I developed the show. I don't know how I even got the idea, but one day while we were talking about my show, I played him one of my old reel-to-reel tapes of the Phone Taps I had recorded just for fun when I first started at POWER.

"Wow, that's funny," Jason said.

So I played him another one.

"Got any more of them?" he asked.

I played him all of what I had. He thought about it for a few minutes.

"I think we need to do something like this on the air," he said.

That was cool with me.

"I can record these phone calls," I said.

That was all that was really involved in doing it. I didn't have loop-to-loop or any other special technology behind them. The phone taps were just phone calls.

Once I started doing the calls with Jason, it just built from there.

When I got people on the phone, they always asked my name.

"Steve Larkiss," I said the first time.

From there, it went to "Steve Luffeigh." I've still got a couple of them recorded from when I was "Steve Luffeigh."

And then, one day, I was talking to this lady.

"And your name is?" she asked.

I don't know what it was, but it just came to me.

"Luther Luffeigh," I said.

It just felt right, like: *Ahhh! That's it! This guy sounds like a Luther Luffeigh.*

"Well how do you spell Luffeigh?" she asked.

I stalled. I couldn't say, "L-O-O-F-A-Y." That sounded fake.

"L-U-F-F-E-I-G-H," I said. "The first F is silent."

Not long after that, I was at the house, and I went to go take a piss. While I was in the bathroom, I thought of the Dr. Dre song *"Got your phone tapped. What you goin' to do?"*

Again, it just felt right, and I thought, *Oh shit.*

I went back into my bedroom and I wrote it on a piece of paper, "Phone Taps."

Then, the next time I went to take a piss, I thought, *Oh I got to loop an instrumental under that.* It all came together in my head, and I knew I had it.

The next morning, I went into the studio and debuted Phone Taps with Luther Luffeigh. Phone taps went through the roof. It was always good to have a couple of signature bits that people liked. Between "Shakin' My Ass", "The Dreidel Song", and Phone Taps, I was riding a good wave. With the pressure I was under in the mornings, I needed everything I had in my arsenal.

19

MORNING OBSESSION

Once I moved to mornings, my stress level went up. I don't remember thinking that it was affecting how much I ate, but I'm pretty sure it did. I think a lot of people go for food when they're stressed out. We have this mentality like we deserve a treat because we're under a lot of pressure, so we have that fast food, or that fatty meal, or that candy bar at the end of the workday when we're fading. As if eating healthy is a punishment. Let me tell you, what all that fatty food does to your body and your health is the punishment. Living to see sixty-five and beyond—which I'm pretty sure I would not have, the way I was going—that's the treat.

I was eating a little bit more in the mornings because I was up and on the air. Then, since I had afternoons and nights off, I was going out to eat, too. I scheduled meetings around food. I stopped for fast food during my drive home from work in the afternoons. While I wasn't going out as much at night because I had to wake up around the same time that I used to get home from the clubs, when I did hit the night-life with my crew, we'd always grab a late night meal on our way home. I didn't notice it at the time, but my whole life revolved around food.

The longer I was at POWER, the more people in Los Angeles knew who I was. And my size was a major part of my personality. We even ran a jingle from Frank V. of the rap group Proper Dos:

"Power, to the 106, from 7:00 to 11:00, Big Boy's in the mix. Spinning them hits that you like. Now who's that 400 pound G. on the mic? Big Boy."

Artists started to put my size in their rhymes. Mack 10 did me a drop where he was talking about hiding guns in rolls of stomach fat because I had told him the story about getting arrested.

And when I did the music videos, it was crazy. The thing with radio is that, no matter how many people listen to a DJ on the air, they don't know what he looks like. But after people saw me on MTV, people knew I was really a big boy.

After I'd been on the morning show for about a year, I did my first billboard. Then, it seemed like anyone who didn't know me suddenly did. I had never thought I'd have a billboard, even once I started at POWER. Not everybody there had one, and I appreciated that it was happening. But I definitely didn't have any idea how colossal it would be.

I could remember when The Baka Boyz billboard first came up a few years before that. I was driving with Nick V. one day when he mentioned it to me.

"Oh, man, our billboard is up," he said.

So we drove over to where it was and parked underneath their billboard and just looked up at it. That was really something. I remember just standing there, seeing my homeboy on top of this huge billboard and just being so happy for him.

Now, fast forward. Suddenly, that was happening to me. When the station first hit me up with the idea, I thought it was amazing. I wasn't even thinking that we had to do something crazy or out of the box that would get everybody talking. I didn't go into it like that. I just thought it would be cool. So then we brainstormed concepts. I think it was the station's marketing director Diana who came up with the Morning Obsession idea. At that time, there were these billboards for Calvin Klein's perfume Obsession that had these models standing there in their whities. So, she wanted to do a billboard that said, "Our models are better than your models," OR "Our models can beat up your models."

That sounded funny, so we got everything set up, and I headed over to where the photo shoot was happening. By this point, I was close to 500 pounds. But that was the crazy thing about me and my weight. Even when I was near my biggest as I was then, I was always comfortable with myself. In fact, after the initial billboard idea was developed, I was the one who took it to the extreme. On the day of the shoot, we had T-shirts and shorts and a bunch of different outfits. But I was thinking about how the Calvin Klein dude, I can't remember if it was Marky Mark or some other cat, was just in his briefs. I figured how could we do a Calvin Klein billboard if I wasn't in my drawers. *Fuck it, I'm doing that shot,* I thought as I arrived at the shoot that day.

If I wasn't so happy in my own skin, there's no way I would have gone with that concept. Even today, after I've lost almost 300 pounds, I wouldn't do those billboards. People have so many pictures of me when I was at my biggest with my shirt off. Back then, I used to flaunt it. I used to pull my shirt off anywhere and everywhere: walking down the hallways at the station, onstage, in front of twenty thousand people at the car show. It didn't matter. I couldn't wait to take my shirt off.

On the day of the shoot, when I walked out in my boxers and no shirt, the people in charge from the station were so excited about how good the billboard was going to be that they lost their minds. I could see on their faces that they were thinking, *Shoot it! Hurry up, before he changes his mind.* They didn't understand how cool I was with how I looked.

In fact, even after the shots were taken, it seemed like they still weren't sure I would really go through with the whole thing. The photos turned out pretty crazy. There were some shots where I was laying down, doing my sexy thing, and it just looked ridiculous. The fat was falling where it wanted to. There was no way I could control that fat. Once I got on my side, it just melted all over me. And remember, this was before Photoshop. I actually had to put a piece of white cloth in my boxers because my big black belly was breaking out through the fly at the front. This was the real deal.

It was crazy, but like I said, I was comfortable. In between shots, I was checking out how the pictures looked—seeing the reality I was about to unveil to the world. I was still walking around the whole time without a robe on. It wasn't like I needed to be covered up as soon as we were done. It wasn't like I felt degraded or exploited. I was having fun. And even when the shoot was over and the pictures were going to print, I never had second thoughts or felt like: *Damn, why did I let them take that picture? Maybe I shouldn't have done that.*

So, we got our shot, and I had my billboard, just like The Baka Boyz. Of course, I didn't know that, in the end, my billboards weren't just billboards. They were a phenomenon. The first time I got clued into what was going down, I was at this club in Hollywood. This dude came up to me and just started laughing.

"Big Boy, man, you a fucking fool," he said. "Man, you're hilarious."

I thought he was talking about something I'd said on the air. I was waiting for him to say whatever had made him laugh.

"I just saw that shit," he said. "You up there in your fucking boxers, man."

"The billboards are up?" I said.

"Yeah, they got this big billboard up on the highway."

"Where?"

"Off Highland."

He told me the cross streets. Just like that, my crew and I left the club so I could go see it with my very own eyes and celebrate my big, beautiful self. We drove over there, to what I think was the intersection at Highland and Franklin in Hollywood—I had prime real estate—and that's when it really hit me. We parked and got out. I just looked up. There were these bright lights shining on it. I couldn't believe it, my billboards were massive.

Oh shit, I thought.

It wasn't something I'd ever been working towards. I was just focused on doing my gig and doing a good job at it. Suddenly, this had happened. The billboards were everywhere. Everybody was talking about them. I honestly never got used to it.

I remember, a little while later, I was coming down Highland, and I got caught at the light. I looked up and was right beneath one of my billboards. Then I looked over to the car at my side. There was this white couple. Just by looking at them, I guessed that they probably didn't listen to my show. The man tapped the lady and caught her attention to look at the billboard. She put her hand over her mouth and started shaking her head and laughing. They were in their car just rolling. I mean their reaction to that billboard was crazy.

These motherfuckers don't even know I'm right next to them, I thought.

After that, people that I never thought would have listened to the station were coming up to me. I was in the store once, and this 60-year-old white man came up to me to talk to me about my billboard. Again and again, I kept hearing the same thing:

"I saw your billboard."

"You know, I never listened to you before, but I saw your billboard and I had to turn you on."

Yeah, this feels crazy, I thought.

I think it was crazy for the listeners, too. A lot of people were surprised to see who Big Boy really was.

"I didn't know you were black," I heard.

Even Queen Latifah was like, "Big Boy, that's you, man? I thought you was Puerto Rican."

Even more than that, I heard, "Man, I did not know you were that big."

This contrasted The Baka Boyz billboards that went up before mine. They always got comments like, "Man, ya'll aren't that big."

But with me, I always heard, "Damn, you are a big boy."

And, "You're like humungous. They shouldn't even call you Big Boy."

Even though I probably felt more comfortable with being fat and naked in front of millions of people than I ever did with all the attention I got for doing it, that was a good moment. I was excited when I drove down the street and saw myself on the side of buildings. It really felt like there was such strong momentum for me. It felt like everything was firing on all cylinders. At that point, music was healthy, revenue was healthy, radio was healthy—and I was right in the thick of it.

Between the billboards and changing up the bits on the show to match the tone of the marketing stuff, the show really picked up. When I started mornings, the show was far from being a top ten-rated show in Los Angeles. Then, within two or three years, we were always in the top three, nonstop. And it's just grown from there: now we're in thirty markets.

20

MAKING IDA PROUD

It wasn't just a big deal to get my own billboard. It was a big deal to get my own billboard in Los Angeles. I had grown up in L.A. To see my face on streets that I had rode the bus down so many times over the years was unbelievable. I'm pretty sure there was a billboard over one of the motels we stayed in. I think that says it all right there.

Then it seemed like everything, good and bad, happened all at once at the end of 1998, and into early 1999. In late 1998, I got the money together to purchase my first house in Sherman Oaks, CA. Around the holidays, I planned to remodel the house and all of that. And then, in early 1999, Mom went into the hospital. Her doctors told us that she was gravely ill and that she wasn't going to make it. She was only fifty-seven, but she had so many things wrong at once—her heart, diabetes, high blood pressure—that any one of those illnesses alone could have killed her. It seemed impossible, but my siblings and I knew that she was going to pass away soon.

The doctors had her in the ICU for about a month. While she was in there, she was on a ventilator. She was very coherent, which was great because my siblings and I were all in there with her, making sure she was comfortable and had everything she needed. But mostly, we were making sure she wasn't alone when her time came. Then, she started breathing better and her doctor wanted to see if she could breathe on her own. We gave him the go ahead.

"Within six hours, if she's not breathing on her own, she can pass," he said.

That was hard to hear. She was still so young; and I don't have to say how much I loved her. But we were there with her, understanding that we were bearing witness to her final hours. It was eerie, how you could have set your watch to this. After five hours, fifty-nine minutes, fifty-nine seconds, as soon as it hit the six-hour mark that she'd been off the ventilator, BAM, she started breathing crazy. We all started to panic because we told the doctors not to put her on a machine to resuscitate her if she started to go. But of course now that she was really going, we couldn't stand to lose her. We called her doctor back in.

"Put her on the machine!" we said. "Put her on the machine!"

All these doctors and nurses were running around, trying to help my Mom. I was sitting down next to her bed, where she was propped up, real high. She was breathing hard, trying to catch her breath. And then, she looked over at me, and she winked at me. That was Ida.

"Okay, you guys need to step out because we've got to do a procedure on her chest," her doctor said.

I could barely make myself leave the room because I didn't know if I would ever see her again, but we all did as we were told. They were able to put her on the machine. They managed to stabilize her. I guess she wasn't ready to go yet. After that, she healed up, and even got out of the hospital. I sent a limousine to pick her up and bring her home.

When she got a little stronger, I called her to make plans to get together.

"Mom, I'm going to pick you up," I said. "What do you want to do?"

"I want to go see your billboards, I want to see your house, and I want to go to Hometown Buffet," she said.

I went to get her, and she was in a wheelchair, so I picked her up out of the chair and loaded her into my Suburban. It was wonderful just having that time to talk with her. We had always had great conversations, but it went deeper now. My sisters Nicole and Sherrille were with us that night, but I hardly remember them being there because the conversation I had with Mom was so intense. I finally asked her things I'd always wanted to know about when she was growing up in Mississippi, and whether it was hard moving to Illinois. And she told me how proud she was of me and how much she appreciated that I had made her life easier. She explained how life had always been hard for her, even as a child.

First, I took her to see the billboards. It was March and it was nighttime, so it was dark. I pulled up on one of my billboards at Ventura and Fulton, and it was huge, lights and everything. There I was. Mom was sitting in the back seat. I rolled down the window for her so she could really see it. She just sat there, looking up at the billboard and then she started laughing.

"My baby is so crazy," she said.

I let her just look at it and marinate on it for a while. Then we drove off. I took her to my new house. I put her in her chair and I rolled her from room to room. I told her about all of the renovations I planned to make. Mostly, I wanted her to see what her son had accomplished and the great work that I felt like she had done to get me to where I was.

Then, she wanted to eat, so I took her to Hometown Buffet. But it was cold that night, and the line was real long. I didn't want her to get sick.

"Mom, I don't want you to go out and get cold," I said. "Can I take you somewhere else?"

"That's alright, baby," she said. "Let's go to Sizzler instead." Mom was always real frugal.

So we went to Sizzler and had a nice time.

"I'll take you to Hometown Buffet next week," I promised.

And then, I drove her home and dropped her off. When I was getting her out of my car, and holding her to put her into her chair, it felt different somehow. It was always special with Mom, but this time I just appreciated her so much and was so grateful for that time with her.

The next week, before I'd had the chance to take her to the Hometown Buffet, she got ill again. She went back into the hospital. She called and left me a message.

"Baby, Mommy's sick," she said. "Mommy's back in the hospital."

And then, she started singing, because she would always call us kids and sing to us, "You are so beautiful."

She died a week later, on March 31, 1999. I was so glad that I had been able to take her to do all of the stuff that she wanted to do. And I knew how proud of me she was. But losing her was the hardest thing I've ever been through. I dealt with it the only way I knew how. She died on a Wednesday. I was back at work on Friday. Not because it didn't hurt. But radio was my therapy. I actually felt bad that my brothers and sisters didn't have that outlet.

It's crazy, though, because to this day, I have never been able to walk into a Hometown Buffet. They even asked me to do a sponsorship at one point. As much as I knew how badly Mom wanted to go, I just couldn't do it. I've never accepted an invitation, a ribbon-cutting, nothing. If I can't go with her, I'm not going to go for the rest of my life.

In Mom's house in Culver City, a bunch of my family stays there—my sisters Sheila, Sherrille, and Nicole, and my brother Keith. My sister Charlene and her kids and her husband stay at my house in Sherman Oaks. We still think of the Culver City place as Mom's house. On every Christmas and Thanksgiving, we gather there. That house is our hub. We do all of our family dinners there.

Now that I'm older and I truly understand it, I'm so grateful for everything Mom did. Some of the best things that I learned in life were just from watching the way she treated people. She was really an open soul. I always knew my mother was someone special. It wasn't like I had to grow up and wait until after she passed to realize how much of a jewel she was. I knew it when she was here with us. Of course, it was when I got older and had a job and kids of my own that I finally realized all of the sacrifices she made. I remember driving home from the station one day after she died, when everything was good in my life, and I started crying.

Now I understand, I thought.

And I really did. I finally got just how hard she had worked and all of the lessons she had tried to teach me over the years. Just like that, I heard her voice in my head and really thought about and felt what a wonderful mother she was. It was beautiful.

21

DON'T TAKE THIS RIDE

1999 was a very hard year for me, but it was impossible not to feel pumped about what was happening with my career. Around this time, I was on vacation in Aruba with my then-girlfriend. I got a call while I was there.

"Hey, this is Harold Austin, the Program Director from THE BEAT," he said. "I just wanted to know if we could talk."

"Harold, you know what, man, I'm in Aruba right now, vacationing," I said. "Why don't you call my agent?"

That was fine with Harold, so I put them in touch. Now, I'm an upfront guy. So I told my boss at POWER that I had gotten a call from THE BEAT. Then, my agent told me that THE BEAT was offering me nearly double what I was currently making at POWER. That was interesting to me. I knew I'd be going through negotiations at POWER at some point. I'd always wondered what I could get paid at THE BEAT. But I liked where I was at. I didn't want to change my world just for money.

"I'm fine," I said to my agent.

This wasn't some sort of hustle to get them to put more money on the table, either. I was good with my place at POWER. I wanted my agent to tell them that. The next day, my agent called me again, this time during a break in my morning show.

"THE BEAT came back with another offer," he said.

"Alright," I said.

"Are you sitting down?" he asked.

"No, but I can," I said.

He told me that THE BEAT had come back with a figure that was *more* than double what I was making at POWER. I looked at the clock: 9:45 am. I still had fifteen minutes left of my show to finish up before I was off the air.

How am I gonna get through my show with this on my head? I thought.

Things got even crazier. Both POWER and THE BEAT were in on the contract talks. They kept going back and forth. THE BEAT was offering me some serious money. If I went to THE BEAT, it would have meant being off the air for three months because of a non-compete clause in my contract with POWER. No problem. THE BEAT was offering to fly me and my crew anywhere we wanted to go for those three months. They were offering me anything and everything I could possibly want: a Mercedes, my own studio, my own offices. Everything we asked for, they were going to give it to us. But POWER was still in the running. They were playing the match game. And, more than that, I always felt like they were family. But THE BEAT would not give up. It finally got to the point where THE BEAT was just throwing so much money and so many other things at me that the negotiations started to get me almost physically sick. My stomach was upset. I couldn't eat. I couldn't sleep. It felt like my mind was constantly racing. I didn't know where to go.

Do I pack up and go to THE BEAT? Do I stay at POWER?

I was really fucked up over the decision. My career wasn't about money. Never had been. And so this whole thing wasn't feeling right.

Finally, I made an announcement to the powers that be at POWER and the people at THE BEAT:

"Give me three days," I said. "Let me think about it for three days. That's all I need. And I'll come back with a decision."

POWER respected my request. They had always let me know that they wanted me there, but they would understand if I needed to leave. Somehow, that felt like family. THE BEAT was letting me know that they wanted me there in a big way. But that just felt like business. Still, it was a big decision and I wanted to be sure.

On the second night, I had a dream. In the dream, I was standing on a dark street and a car pulled up. The back door opened. I got in the back seat and closed the door. There were two people in the front seat who were both wearing hoods. Before we drove off, someone walked in front of the car. I realized it was the Grim Reaper. *Dude, that's symbolic of death,* I thought.

Then, as the car drove off, the person in the passenger seat took her hood off and turned around. It was Mom. She was shaking her head, like, *Don't take this ride. Don't do it.* I reached up to remove the hood from the person that was driving the car. It was Steve Smith, the guy who had been brokering the deal and trying to get me over to THE BEAT.

When I woke up, Craig Wilbraham had Steve Smith on the phone with me.

"Yo," I said.

"It's three days," Craig said.

"Yeah, I know Craig," I said. "But I'm in the same place."

They were going over all of the things they were going to give me again and saying that if I signed the deal that day, they'd send a Mercedes Benz to my house that was just like Craig's car, which I had complimented at one of our earlier meetings.

He was really selling it to me and greed was stirring inside of me.

"Big Boy, I think this is a great move for you," he said. "Think about how proud your mother would be."

My mom had just died a few months earlier.

"What the fuck did you just say to me?" I said.

"Oh, I said think about how proud your mother would be," he said again.

"Man, my mother just died," I said.

"I know, I know," he said. "My mother just died also. I was just saying how proud she would be."

"Man, don't you ever bring my mother into some motherfucking negotiation," I said. "I don't even want to talk to you."

As I started to hang up the phone, I could hear his voice.

"Big, Big, Big."

"Hello?" I said.

"Yeah, do I still have a shot?" he said.

I didn't say anything else. I just hung the phone up on him. As soon as my dial tone cleared, I called POWER and said I was ready to sign. I knew right then that my dream had been right. THE BEAT was the car; the Grim Reaper was Craig Wilbraham. Steve Smith was in the driver seat. Mom was telling me not to take that ride.

After that, the guys at THE BEAT went and got The Baka Boyz, Nautica de la Cruz, and a dude who was a writer for my show. THE BEAT's management thought they were taking down POWER. And they were throwing the money around. I didn't care. I was happy with my decision. And then, once all of those people got over to THE BEAT, the powers that be sold the station, and all those people got moved around or fired.

My intuition always lets me end up right where I'm supposed to be.

22

THE SPLITS

My first billboard had gotten everyone talking and tuning into the show. Now we needed to do another one that was just as bold. We came up with some wild ideas. There was one where I was dressed as a Playboy Bunny, with the ears. That was almost as much a hit as the first Morning Obsession billboard.

"You're fucking crazy," people said.

I was, because under that little outfit, I was completely naked. And let's just say that my size wasn't exactly getting smaller.

We did Spider-Man. We did one that was a play on the Marlboro Man cigarette ads.

In each and every one of them, I was huge. And in most cases, my size was a part of the joke. But when I look back at those billboards, there's not one that I'm embarrassed of or where I feel like I played myself.

Though I was completely comfortable with my physique, not everyone else was. Somebody called the station and complained about the billboard with the bunny ears because it was right outside his office, and he didn't want to look at it.

One time a woman I met tried to tell me that POWER was exploiting me with the billboards. I had to explain to her that the billboards were my idea. This was who I was. Nobody was telling me to do anything. She got it then. And I wasn't just trying to make myself feel better. I knew where my boundaries were. After I did the Spider Man billboard, one of my bosses had what she thought was a brilliant idea.

"We're doing the POWER staff meeting," she said. "Can you wear the Spider Man costume to the meeting?"

Hell fucking no, I thought. *That's beneath me.*

I said it a little more politely than that, but it was a definite *N-O*.

I've always been a person where there is nothing that someone can make me do. It's not because I'm Big Boy in the morning. I've always been like that. The way I figure it, I'm a black man first. I've always had a fun personality and a good time, but I'm not going to dance and shuck and jive because someone wants me to.

Other than those few little incidents, everything was love. Everything was very, very positive. I think people could see that even though I was big, I was happy. I was confident. If the first billboard had been popular, now they were really everywhere. Sometimes I'd be driving, and I'd be damn near back-to-back, like I was seeing myself on every freeway I was driving.

It was clear that more and more people were tuning in as a direct result of the billboards. Even guests on the show started to talk about them. I'd open the door and the person would walk in laughing before we even started talking.

"Man, you're a fool." Or, "Man, I saw your billboard."

And after that, our conversation would go from zero to sixty in a matter of seconds because it was like we were already old friends by the time I asked the first question.

Then, I did a billboard that created almost as big of a sensation as the original Morning Obsession billboards. It was one that showed me doing a split. Like I said, I've been able to do the splits since I was a kid. But seeing a little kid do a split is one thing. It's another thing altogether to see a 500-pound man do a split. People could not believe that was me in the picture. They were sure it was photoshopped somehow. But it was me, alright. The crazy story, though, was that the photos they used were originally just going to be a tester. I did the split, and they took some test photos. I held my hands up for the last three test shots: click, click, click. I was supposed to come back and shoot the rest of the billboard. But, then, I fell in the shower and hurt my groin. I couldn't do the splits for a while. So they just used what we already had; and that became the billboard.

As soon as it went up, I never heard the end of it.

"Okay, man, now how did they do that?" people asked me.

"No, that's me," I said.

"Man, get the fuck out of here."

That billboard had another kind of payoff that I hadn't ever imagined. Right after it went up, I was hanging with Dr. Dre, shooting a video for the Xzibit song "Year 2000," which Dre had produced. We were at this big house with something like 2000 acres of land, so they could land a helicopter and do all of this other stuff. Everybody was sitting around talking.

"Hey, Big, what did they do for you to do the splits?" Dre asked. "How did they do that computer-wise?"

"Man, that's me," I said.

"Man, get the fuck out of here."

"No, man, Dre, really that's me."

Fuzz rolled up, and as he and I had already done to other people, he cosigned Dre in order to set what happened next in motion.

"Man, that's not him," Fuzz said.

"Dre, trust me man, it's me." I said.

"Do it right now," Dre said.

"Dre, I'm not gonna do it right now," I said. "You put some money up, I'll do it."

He was looking at me, really looking at me, to see if I was serious.

"Fuck no, that's not you," he said.

So then, Phillip Atwell, who was directing the Dre shoot came in, and he didn't believe it either. He thought he knew how they'd faked it with the computer.

"Man, nah," he said. "That's not real."

"Phillip, no man, that is me," I said. "If you bet, I'll take your money."

So Dre put up $2,000 and Phillip put up $2,000.

"Come on let's step over here," I said, because I didn't want to let everyone see what I was truly capable of and ruin the opportunity for future bets.

We stepped over to a secluded area of the house. I kicked my shoes off because I always try to do the splits barefoot so I can go down more smoothly. Dre, Phillip, and a few of the homeys were standing there. Fuzzy was holding the money.

"No, Big, you got to put yours up too," they said.

"I don't have to put it up," I said. "I'm taking this money home with me."

First I made it look like I was struggling, which they totally bought. And then BAM, I went down, just like that, looking at them the whole time, and did a split. They just lost it. They were running in every direction, slapping their hands. I mean, Dre, the look on his face could have been an album cover. He was blown away.

"Oh my God!" Phillip said. "It was worth my $2,000 just to see that."

I picked up the money, and I was cool. But I heard about it all that day, because they still couldn't believe it. And then, later on that same night—literally not even five hours later—I got into a conversation with Snoop about it.

"Oh, cuz, nah that's not you," Snoop said.

"No, that's me," I said. "Put your money up."

Snoop was ready to go. We were at the shoot for this TV show called *Farm Club*. They were filming the N.W.A. reunion. Cube and a bunch of other cats were there. I had already gotten Cube with the same trick. Dre was there, and of course he knew what I could do. Later in the night, Dre must have heard Snoop talking into his mic about me and whether or not I could do the splits. Next thing I knew, Dre came over the speaker.

"Nah, Snoop don't do that shit, he's trying to get you," Dre said. "That motherfucker got us for like four Gs today."

So I never got Snoop because Dre blocked it. But I got Dre. I got Cube. I'd actually been getting people for years. I remember making the guys in The Pharcyde put up $50 because they couldn't believe I could do the splits, back when we were on tour together. But when the billboard came out, it took it to the next level. I got some people in the studio, too. It was a joke for probably six months, until word got out and no one would bet me. But, before that, off the billboard alone, I made at least $20,000 to $25,000. After that, people believed I could do the splits.

23

BIG-BONED

Everybody was talking about the billboards, about how crazy it was that I was up there, as fat as I was, half-naked, doing the splits for everyone to see. There was no denying just how big this Big Boy could be.

But what's really wild is that, this whole time, no one in my life said anything to me about my weight or what it might be doing to my health. Maybe it's because a lot of my crew worked for me at POWER and they were used to thinking of me as the boss. Or maybe that's just how people knew me and they were used to it. Whatever it was, no one said a word. Sure I had some big homeys who told me about their own diets. And I had some cats that tried to get me to go to the gym with them. But I had a trainer. I worked out. I was actually in pretty good shape, considering my size. I was just humungous. I blew off any suggestions that I had a serious health problem.

But I have to admit, it impacted my life each and every day. When cats were wearing football jerseys, I couldn't fit into them. And then, by the time I lost the weight, they were out of style. I always kept myself clean and spiffy, but I still wanted to wear what other people were into.

I was steadily gaining weight throughout these years. With me, I could put on 10 pounds and it would just disappear on my frame. I wasn't stepping on scales all the time, either. The way I noticed I was gaining weight was by my clothes. I remember putting on a shirt and realizing it was too small.

Oh shit, I've got to move to a 6X.

And I wasn't crying about it. I just bought a 6X and that was that.

At my biggest I was an 8X. And I had 10X shirts in the house, just in case.

But there's no 10X Sean John shirt. So being the size I was, it kept me out of name brands. I had to buy whatever I could buy. When my brother got married, I had the hardest time finding a tuxedo. We damn near had to change what the groomsmen wore because they had to accommodate me.

I'd always seen cats wearing crew jackets for their show or their movie. I wanted to get leather jackets made for everyone in *the Neighborhood*. But when I started looking around, they didn't have my size. Not only that, there was no pattern for my jacket because I was so big. Finally, I found a guy who could do it, but he had to do what he could for mine. Then, he made everyone else's jacket to match.

When I finally got my jacket, I was so excited. It was my first leather jacket because I'd never been able to find a leather jacket in my size before. I brought it home, put it in the closet, and it broke the hanger. And when I traveled, it damn near needed its own suitcase because it was so big and heavy. Somehow I didn't trip out on that, though. The same thing happened when I was folding up my size 66 pants and putting them in my luggage. It didn't phase me. At least that's what I would have said if you'd asked me about it back then. I never told anyone, but when I traveled I would stand there at the baggage claim, just praying that my bag was there. If they had lost my luggage, I was in trouble. Where was I going to go buy some new size 66 pants? Where was I going to go get an 8X shirt?

I avoided movies, too. I had to see movies in West Wood because either I couldn't get into the movie theater-sized seat—or I could, but it was just too tight and I didn't want to be stared at. Today, most theaters have stadium seating because we all got so damn big. But with a regular movie theater chair, the arms only went so far on either side. I would kind of squeeze myself in and try to sit back, but both arms would just dig into my fat. So when I went to a movie or a concert, I made sure I got the aisle seat, in order to spread out as much as possible.

It got to where I set up my life to accommodate moments like this; and when I didn't feel like dealing with it, I stayed home. Essentially, my whole life and everything I did was dictated by my size. But at the time, I just clowned about it and acted like it rolled off me. But it got to me sometimes. It wasn't like I was just oblivious and living in la-la land. It's just that I was too comfortable in my skin—and too used to my way of living—to admit that my weight was going to kill me. Here I was, morbidly obese, in denial, living it up and not doing anything about it.

I tried to tell myself that I was staying home because I just wanted to chill. But it got inside of me. I was still basically a happy person. But I was now aware of my weight, of what it stopped me from doing and how I had to account for it in other ways. I couldn't comfortably fit in a car, so I drove a big truck. When I flew on Southwest Airlines, where they board the flights according to first come first serve, I made sure I got there early. That way, I boarded the plane first and got myself squeezed into my two seats—I couldn't fit in just one, and I couldn't tear myself in half, so I had to buy two. Otherwise, I didn't know if I would be able to find a seat where I fit. But that was just the way I rolled. When I didn't make it there early, and I had to board the plane after people were already on, I was very self-conscious about the looks people gave me as they saw me walking down the aisle towards them. Even though I was as big as I was, I can look at somebody now, and maybe they're like 325 pounds, and think *Oh, wow* when I see them coming towards me on an airplane. And then I give myself a reality check. *Dude, I was, like, 175 pounds bigger than that person. So what did I look like coming down that aisle?*

To most people, I wasn't the biggest person that they'd seen that day at the airport. I was the biggest person they'd seen in their lives. And I could feel it just radiating off people as I passed by them.

Okay, who am I gonna sit next to? I wondered, looking for a kind face in the crowd.

Even once I was in my seat, I couldn't put the tray table down. I couldn't put the seatbelt on without a seatbelt extension. When I sat down, I was so big that my thighs automatically hit the recline button, and I'd go backwards without meaning to. It used to be that I'd have to worry about that happening the whole flight. And then, I got the idea to make what I called sky caps. This was a bottle cap that I put right over the button, so my thigh could hit it without pushing down the seat recline button. I always made sure I had a bottle cap in my carry on when I flew.

I was Big Boy; so I always found workarounds. Often, I traveled with my crew. I remember, one time, we all flew out of Phoenix. It was Fuzzy and me, and my homeboy, Imani, who's a thin dude. When we got on the plane, we pointed him to the seat between Fuzzy and I.

"You've got to sit right there," I said.

"Dude, that seat doesn't even exist," he said.

Somehow, he got in there between us, but this dude's arm was damn near above his head, just trying to accommodate our size on either side of him.

There were times when my whole crew flew coach and I had to fly first class, because it was the only way the seats were big enough for me. For awhile, I had that written into all of my contracts, that if I got flown somewhere, it had to be first class. Then, it got to the point where I bought both seats, even in first class, so I didn't have to deal with the humiliation anymore. Even up until recently, HBO still sent me two seats when they flew me somewhere to do something for them because it was written into the original deal that we signed.

It even got to where my size, and the size of a lot of guys in my crew, determined where we ate. We called ahead before going to a restaurant.

"Do they have fat man chairs in there?" we asked.

Or we had one of my cats jump out and run into a restaurant to do recon.

"Man, see if it's fat friendly in there."

It was a necessity. If the restaurant had booths, I couldn't fit in them. If we went somewhere and they had arms on the chair, I couldn't sit down and eat.

The same thing went for when I was broadcasting from somewhere. I'm sure my producer Jason had to make sure they accommodated my size more times then I knew. I was too big to sit on standard plastic and metal chairs. And, with a lot of chairs, I had to be conscious and make sure I didn't break them. That was just the way it was. That was my norm.

I was good at getting by, but there were moments that got through to me and hurt. I could sit here all day and say: "Oh, man, you know, I didn't really trip off of it." The truth is that there's no great feeling that I could have gotten, walking around at 500 pounds, and seeing how people responded to me.

I was in Paris one time, and I turned around to see a guy and his wife videotaping me. When they caught me looking at them, they tried to play like they weren't treating me like a freak, but it was obvious what they were up to.

And people could be rude without even realizing it.

"How do you wipe your ass?" one dude asked me.

"Man, how do you have sex?" another dude asked me one time.

My ex, whom I dated for seven years, told me that her play-cousin, R&B artist Marques Houston, asked her the same thing. And without getting too graphic here, let's just say that my body was crazy by that point, so this was something else that I had to accommodate, too. Because my stomach hung down so low, I had to hold my stomach up or get into a certain position to have intercourse. But again, that was just my life. I knew I was fat. It wasn't like I didn't know. But I got on with it. I know it's hard to believe how I was living. Looking back, I feel the same kind of doubt.

If I can say that about her, and feel like she's in denial, then I must have been in denial too—about my emotional eating, about how it was making me fatter and fatter, about how I felt about being fat. I think we all experience denial about the things that we know we should change or improve, but we can't always seem to get a handle on them. To avoid our own denial, we create some collective denial with our family members and our friends. Just like my mom never made the connection between how much and what kind of food she was feeding me, and what it was doing to my weight. Or, how I surrounded myself with other cats who ate as much as I did. My denial wasn't anything they weren't dealing with themselves. This made it harder for anyone to confront me about my weight and tell me how it was impacting my health.

Like I've said time and again, though, I mostly felt happy. If there was one button that said 500 pounds and another that said 190 pounds, I would have pushed the 190 pound button. So, maybe I felt happy; but I knew I could be happier. And the reason I could hold both of those feelings inside of me, I think, went back to my childhood. When we were broke, I was happy. When we were homeless, I was happy. But when we had a home, or when money was okay, I was happier.

I don't know if it was just a fog that was over me. Or maybe I felt like all this fat was just the way it was. This was just me. That big-boned shit—I really believed it. I was 133 pounds in the fourth grade. I never thought I could be a regular size.

And nothing seemed able to shake me—not even when I got to be bigger than Human Beat Box from The Fat Boys, who had died at age 28 in 1995, weighing 450 pounds. Not even after losing my mom in 1999, when she was only fifty-seven. Granted, my mom was never obese, she was just mommy-fat. But when she passed on, it was from everything that could go wrong in a body after a lifetime of not eating right.

And then, in 2000, Big Pun died of a heart attack at age 28. That hit me because I had known Pun since he first started coming through L.A.. I'd watched his career take off. Even more than that, he and I had talked about the difficulties of being overweight. Like me, his fat had pushed against the recline button on his seat too many times when he flew. I suggested he use sky caps, and he did. It was like we had a fat man underground network where we traded tips.

In the year before he died, I'd noticed that when he came out to L.A., he was bigger and bigger and bigger. And he was slowing down. One night, I went out to a Pun concert, and I watched backstage as they drove him up on a motorized cart. They had a seat waiting for him to sit down before he got onstage because he was exhausted from walking up the few stairs to the stage.

Pun was bigger than me—I think before he passed, his weight was almost 700 pounds. But when I first met him, there was no way in the world that he was bigger than me. When he surpassed me in size, that hit me. It was one of those things where, when I saw how winded he was at his show, my thought was, *Dude, I need to start exercising.* And then, a few songs later, I thought, *I want to go to IHOP when I get out of here tonight.* Both the thought and the good intention were gone. And the next day, I was right back to my same old patterns.

After Pun's death, Fat Joe called me to go on the air and talk about Pun. He was devastated. It had opened his eyes, too. We talked on the show about obesity and the negative impact it has on one's health.

"Big Boy, we need to take care of ourselves," Joe said. "We can die."

In that moment, I was really invested in what was going on. Pun had passed. I had his Terror Squad leader on the phone. We were both obese. We'd just lost an obese partner of ours, somebody that I had a personal tie to. Every word rung true. I got back to the trainer. The only problem was this—it was enough to spark maybe a month of better living on my part. But a lifetime? Not at all. I was conscious that I was unhealthy, but I wasn't doing anything about it for the long-term.

It was always: *Oh, I'll start on Monday. Oh, no, I messed up. It's Wednesday. I'll start again on Monday.* How many Mondays did I think I was going to get?

I knew I was unhealthy. I don't know if I waived it off because I didn't feel like getting a handle on it was realistic. Let's be honest, how many people can really lose 300 pounds? It was almost like it was just easier to stay 500 pounds, even though I knew it was a death sentence.

So even with friends and colleagues passing—even ones who were younger, and 100 to 200 pounds smaller—I still put off getting healthy. I still thought: *That can't happen to me.* At the same time, I could look at somebody who weighed less than me and think: *Man, how did they let themselves go like that?*

In other words, I could be one of the most judgmental and preju- diced severely morbid obese motherfuckers you'd ever met in your life.

There was one person who tried to talk to me about my weight around this time: the Boxer Fernando Vargas. I'd known him for years. He'd always been such a good dude. When I really started getting big, Fernando got concerned enough for me that he finally brought it up. We were on the phone one day, just making small talk and catching up. Then, he started talking about how he comes from a family of big people, about how he's seen how hard it can be and what it can do.

"Big, have you ever thought about surgery or anything like that?" he asked.

"Nah, man," I said. "I'm cool."

"You know, I'll put up some money to pay for it," he said.

I didn't get defensive or anything like that because I knew it came from a place of love. But I wasn't ready to hear it. I let his words slide right off me. It was easy enough to do because I was still avoiding any real self-reflection about my eating, or the possibility that it had gotten out of control for reasons that I wasn't ready to admit. No one else in my life ever mentioned my size to me. As always, my family loved me, no matter what. And I was so used to being Big Boy—at Power 106 and in my personal life—that I radiated the kind of authority that didn't allow people to question me or my lifestyle, even if to do so would have been an act of love. It was going to take someone or something even bigger than Big Boy to make me change.

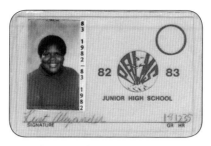

Even the year after I went gangsta, I still cleaned up nice for my school ID photo in eighth grade. My mom Ida wouldn't have had it any other way.

Wearing black may have a slimming effect, but there was only so much it could do by the time my senior class pictures rolled around.

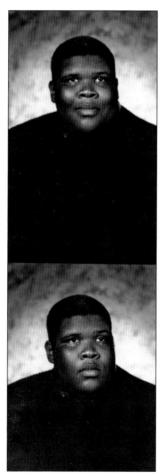

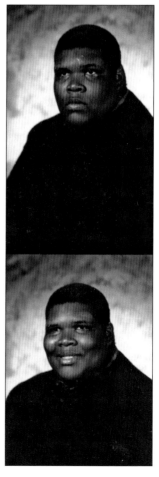

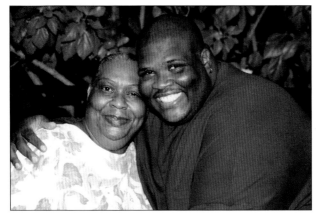

With my mom, Ida, who inspired me to get my Ida's Son tattoo and name my business and charity Ida's Son. Buying her a house was one of the proudest moments in my life.

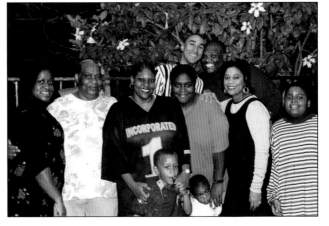

We are Family. For years, my family was all that I needed in the world. Here I am with most of my family unit, from L to R: Charlene, my mom Ida, Nicole, Sherrille, Sheila, my nephew Ian, back row: Kenneth, Big, front row: my nephews, Khody and Khoury.

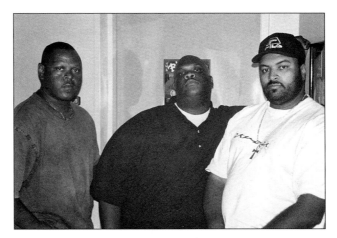

Roger Clayton, the guy who brought Run DMC to my house and told me which turntables to buy when I first started to DJ, me and The Egyptian Lover.

Old School hang with Run DMC, who I first met as a teenager, when Jam Master Jay was still with us.

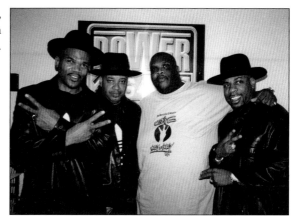

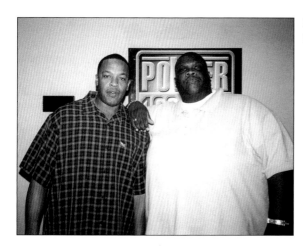

Hanging at the station with Dr. Dre after he did the show.

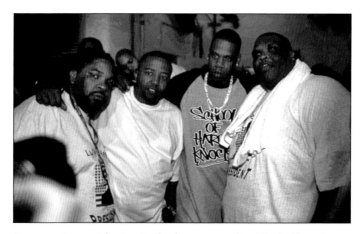

Representing with Jay-Z backstage at the 2000 Powerhouse Concert. Notice my Luther Luffeigh for President T-shirt. *Photo by Zach Cordner*

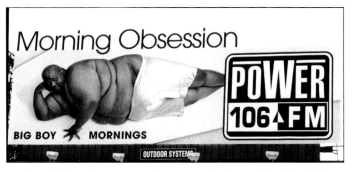

My first billboard, Morning Obsession, which people still talk about today. At the time, I heard: "Man, I did not know you were that big."

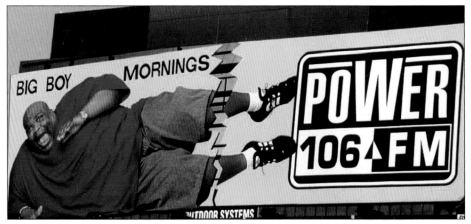

After Morning Obsession madness, we kept Los Angeles laughing with billboard after billboard. Here's one of the later ones.

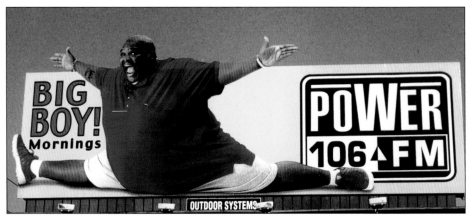

Many have lost money betting a 500 pound guy couldn't do this. But this is all real.

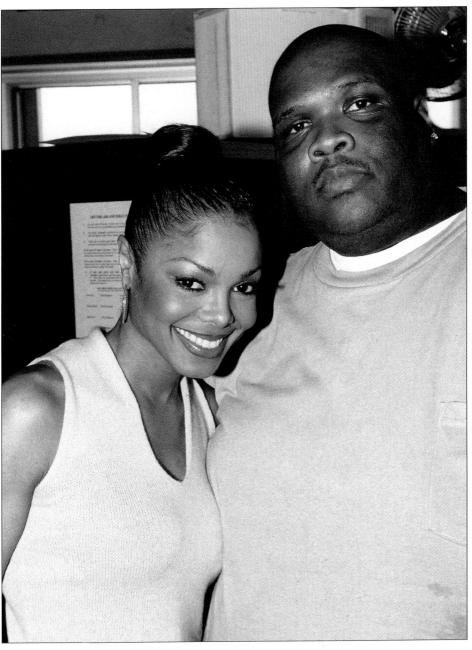

In the studio with Janet Jackson.

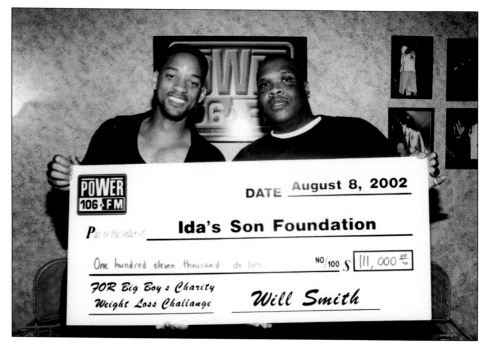

With Will Smith the day he presented me with a check for $111,000 for the 111 pounds he inspired me to lose during my charity weight loss challenge in 2002. I'll always be grateful that he called me out on my weight when no one else would.

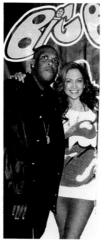

With Jennifer Lopez at the Backstage Breakfast, post-surgery. This was the day I accidentally cut the cord to my protein pack and nearly died, but I would not go to the hospital because the show must go on.

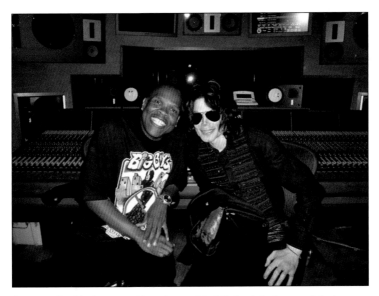

A career highlight, spending time with Michael Jackson while he was working with my old friend will.i.am of The Black Eyed Peas on the 25th anniversary edition of *Thriller* in Las Vegas in January 2008. *Photo by Joel Marasigan*

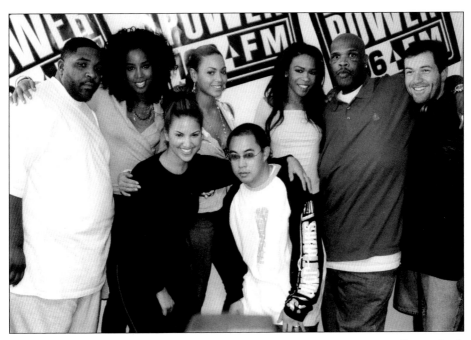

Destiny's Child stops by *The Neighborhood*, (standing, left to right) Fuzzy, Kelly Rowland, Beyonce, Michelle Williams, Big Boy, Jason Ryan, (front) Liz Hernandez, DJ E-Man.

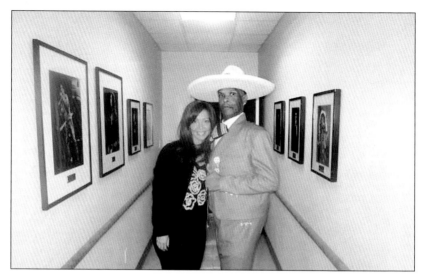

Backstage with my best friend, my wife Veronica, before having one of my bucket list—and most nerve wracking—moments, singing with the great Vicente Fernandez onstage at the Gibson Amphitheater in November 2010.

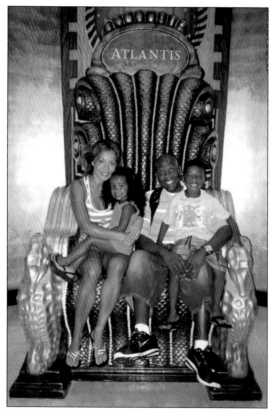

Now, I've got my own family to live for: my beautiful wife Veronica, our daughter Jaide and our son Jayden. Here we are on vacation.

All photos used with the permission of the author and Power 106, unless otherwise specified.

24

THESE ARE THE PEOPLE
IN *THE NEIGHBORHOOD*

In 2001, *the Neighborhood* started taking shape into the show that people have known and tuned into for the past decade, with the likes of Fuzzy Fantabulous, Luscious Liz and Tattoo.

As I've said, William "Fuzzy Fantabulous" West and I go back to the Pharcyde days. I brought him to POWER with me from day one. At first, he came in just to lend a hand, but he ended up making his way onto the air from time to time. Fuzzy was always my funny guy, and for so many years, I delivered my show to Fuzzy. It was like I knew that if I could make Fuzzy laugh, then I knew listeners were laughing, too. In a way, he's been like my meter on the show. He plays a hell of a part in what I do in the day.

Growing up in the church, and in a household with no secular music, Fuzzy had to learn about hip hop when he got older. I was the one who took Fuzzy to his first hip hop club. When I did, he wore dress shoes, slacks and a dress shirt, tucked in. He had a flat top with a pretty little part in it. I was the first one who put a gun in his hand. Back then, he used to wear glasses, before he went and got corrective surgery. I can remember how, behind those lenses, his eyes were open so wide from soaking up all the new stuff he was seeing at that time.

Since then, Fuzzy has lived a lot. I've seen him go from a bald head to dreads. I remember when he moved to New York, and you could not tell him he was not a native. He's lived a lot on the air-waves, too. Once, when he had a hemorrhoid, we had a hemorrhoid nurse come down and open up his butt crack and do the hemor-rhoid test live on the air. I'd say our listeners have really come to know Fuzzy inside and out over the years. But one thing they might not know is that when Fuzzy gets pulled over by the police, or he gets nervous, he passes gas. So if you're around Fuzzy, and you smell something, that's what it is.

The next cat to join our crew came around because of The Hat of Forbidden Questions. After years of doing interviews, I had gotten tired of always asking guests the typical questions about when their next album was coming out. We decided to dig a little deeper. We had a green hat in the studio, and we filled it with questions that the guest had to choose randomly. The object was for the questions to be so hard, or so intrusive, that the guest wouldn't be able to answer and would have to tap out. When word of the hat got around, all of my guests wanted to be the one to answer the most questions before tapping out. It became this macho, braggadocio thing. Snoop had answered six before he tapped out. Everyone wanted to beat that record.

One morning in May 2001, we had Shaq on. We were talking and clowning, and then it was time for The Hat of Forbidden Questions. We built it up; then I held out the hat. Shaq reached in and pulled out a question. It said:

"Have you ever had sex with anyone famous?"

"Yes," Shaq said. "How many do you want me to name?"

This was gonna be good.

"Three," Fuzzy said.

Shaq thought about it for a second, and then he went there.

"Aaliyah, Venus Williams, Cindy Crawford," Shaq said.

This went everywhere. While Shaq was still in the studio with us, Venus was already texting him, "That's fucked up. I can't believe you're blowing me up like that." She later came out and said that she'd only met him once, at a Lakers' game. Shaq ended up saying that he'd made the whole thing up and went on to send letters of apology to all three women. But it took awhile for that part of the story to get out, so everyone thought what he said was true. To this day, I still feel that what he said was true, that when he changed his story, he was just doing damage control. Black listeners were tripping over the fact that he named Aaliyah and Venus. The rest of America was tripping over Cindy Crawford. Other media outlets were calling us and asking us questions about it. I remember being in line at the grocery store during this time. The story was on the cover of *Star* and the *National Enquirer*.

We took it and ran with it.

We had tickets for an upcoming Lakers game, and we announced that we would give those tickets away to one lucky listener who was willing to get a little ink for us. All he had to do was get a tattoo on his forehead that said: I slept with Shaq.

Well, this went off. I don't know if people were doubling up faxes and calls, but we got 800 responses. We picked this one guy, David Gonzalez. He came down to the studio with his girl. He had never been to a great basketball game before, and he wanted to do it. We got him on the air and made sure he was really down.

"I want to do it," he said.

So, boom, we tattooed his forehead and sent him to the game. And from the first time he came around, I saw a character in this guy. I started calling him Tattoo, and he ended up being a regular part of the show. He earned his place in a major way. For a while there, Tattoo was like my Fuzzy, the guy that I played to on the air because I knew that if I could make Tatt laugh, then people out there were laughing, too.

Around that same time in 2001, we were looking for someone to read the news in the morning. That's when we brought in Luscious Liz. Truth be told, when she first came in and I heard her do the news, I didn't like Liz. It wasn't that I didn't like her personally. I just thought she didn't do a good job. But it wasn't like we had a whole wishing well of talent we could pull from. She was the best announcer that we tried out. And Jason heard something in her that I didn't hear at first, so he encouraged me to give her a try. Of course, he was right. Liz was an important part of *the Neighborhood* for ten years.

The funny thing about Liz being on POWER is that she can't dance to save her life. If you see her out on the dance floor, make sure you get out of the way. I have yet to find out what she's dancing to. What she is good at is nutrition, and this has been a big help to me over the years. Liz was the dietician of *the Neighborhood*. She was always bringing in healthy food. She's a salad girl, so she would bring that in. Or, she'd bring in all different kinds of oatmeal. A lot of times, she was the first person to turn me onto a new dish—not all of them healthy. She introduced me to bacon wrapped around a date with crumbled blue cheese inside. That one I didn't like too much, actually. I can remember that Tattoo and I both pretended it tasted good to spare Liz's feelings, while we were looking at each other like, "What is this shit?" But the truth always comes out eventually. Liz would never come in with a plate of enchiladas with grease running all over it. She wouldn't come in with a burger. Instead, she'd have me eat some grass and tree bark. She's never been afraid to lay it down, either. She'd come up to me and say, "You shouldn't be eating that."

As most listeners could probably tell, Liz is a sweetheart. What's surprising about her is that she isn't married. She doesn't have that guy yet. You would have thought that somebody would have locked that up already. A beautiful girl like that, who cooks very well, speaks highly of her mother and father, is very family-driven, and is just a good individual—that's a catch. She did have a high school sweetheart that she dated for ten-plus years. Now, they're the best of friends. But there's no new guy in the picture.

Liz added that female perspective, which was good—especially when all of us dudes in *the Neighborhood* got to talking about something. We definitely benefited from having a woman around. Otherwise, it could have become all locker room. We didn't need just any woman, but a woman like Liz who represented the ladies at home who can't turn on the mic and have their say. When we got to topics like "Who cheats more, men or women?"—or "Why do mean cheat?"—we needed a woman's opinion to liven up the conversation. Any relationship topic we mention always goes through the roof. Everyone has something to say. And everyone is an expert. I think listeners like these topics, too, because we make it personal. I always have my place in the conversation because my ex cheated on me. And Liz had her place because an ex cheated on her. And so people know I've got a personal investment in it when I put forth an opinion, like women cheat better, but not as often—or women cheat for emotional reasons, and men cheat for sex.

Some of the best conversations we've had over the years, which have really gotten listeners going, have been sparked by the big celebrity scandals. The Tiger Woods thing fueled the fire for a long time. Nobody, not even the fellows in *The Neighborhood,* were sticking up for Tiger. We all felt like he'd lost his player stripes; so we talked about that a lot. Other times, it was just Liz saying he was an asshole. Or, we'd talk about how maybe once is permitted. Not only did he not do it once, however, he also made it worse by playing that smiley character the whole time. Personally, I thought that he was a piece of shit; I couldn't even put myself in a position to play devil's advocate for him. There wasn't even much to find funny. My take was more like, *Man, you really scraped your knuckles going to the bottom of that barrel.* But it made for good radio.

More recently, we've talked about U.S. Representative Anthony Weiner, and how more people are getting caught cheating through Facebook or Twitter. That's another one that got people going. We've heard it all:

He sent a message to me by accident.

He pocket dialed and I heard him talking to another girl.

That has led us to talk about how it used to be that a person had to at least call you to tell you when it's over. Now, it's like you've got to vibrate and read that shit as a text. Or it's a direct message over Twitter and they've only got 140 characters to break your heart. So we'll ask listeners to let us know if they've ever been broken up with by text, or things like that. Those topics always make for good shows. I like giving listeners a chance to get in on the talk, too. Lord knows we've all been through it.

Pretty much any celebrity in the news who's dipping out can get a conversation started. There's always someone. That always strikes a chord with listeners because I can guarantee you that somebody right now is having that problem. Also popular is any survey—say, *the top ten hottest girls in the business right now*—because there's always plenty of room for debate. We always end up creating our own list. So, the things that come up in *the Neighborhood* as topics of conversation happen pretty organically. It seems to work out well that way.

It's always been a good vibe in *the Neighborhood* because we all get along. We have a routine that works well for us. We prep the day before and select the phone tap. Then we touch base with each other the night before, so we know what we're going to cover and how the show is going to go. We try to get to the studio a half hour before we start. Once there, we're ready to go, and we take off at full speed. With radio, we have no warm up options—as soon as the mic is turned on, we've got to be running at plus ten already. The last thing we do is grab the day's news. Then, we roll. It's planned spontaneity—and it's a lot of fun. I think listeners can hear that.

25

WILL SMITH GIVES ME A
WEIGHT LOSS CHALLENGE

In late 2001, someone finally broke through my denial about the way I'd been living and what it was doing to my health. It was just like any other day at the show. Will Smith was on as a guest, promoting his film, "Wild, Wild West." He was always a great interview because he was smart and funny. Listeners loved him. We had fun while we talked and everything was good.

After we finished on the air, Will and I left the studio and hung out in the POWER offices. He was wearing a black velour sweatsuit with a muscle tee. He sat on a desk with one leg up, one leg dangling, while I stood nearby talking to him.

"Big," he began. "How old are you?"

"I'm thirty-two," I said. I remember thinking that Will was only one year older than me.

"Man," he said. "You ever thought about, you know, taking some pounds off?"

"Yeah, you know," I said.

I was cool, but I didn't exactly feel great about having him bring it up like that, either. I hoped that if I kind of dodged the subject, he'd let it go.

"But what about your heart?" he said. "You've got to take care of yourself."

For some reason, I heard that.

Damn, what about my heart? I thought.

Suddenly, nothing else existed around me. I didn't know if there was music being played in the office, or if my crew was around. It was like we were in a movie. Everything just blanked out. Will and I were the only people around.

"Well, why don't we do something fun?" he said. "Why don't we do a weight loss challenge and donate the money to charity? I'll give you $1,000 per pound."

I really heard that. I was thinking, *Okay, this is Will Smith. It's charity. I'll lose some weight. I'll get some publicity.* I have to admit that, at first, I was more about having Will Smith as a regular guest on the show than getting my health together. But it was more than that, too. Will is just one of those guys who's always positive, always happy. It meant something to me that he was voluntarily reaching out to me like that. Somehow, I knew that this could maybe work.

Will had to go finish promoting his movie. Then, he was going away with his family for a Christmas vacation. But he was serious about this.

"When I come back in January, let's start it up," he said.

"Alright, I'm in, man," I said.

So Will Smith and I kicked off the weight loss challenge on the show in January of 2002, just like we had agreed. Even though I'd never successfully dieted in my whole life—I'd always fallen victim to the, "I'll start again on Monday" mentality—once I got in it, I was in it. Good thing, too, because everybody was watching me. We talked about it on the show. We kicked it off on the local TV stations, KTLA and Fox. They had cameras in the studio for my initial weigh in. My trainer at the time was named Rod. He brought in his scale that went up to 600 pounds. I didn't know what the number was going to be; but I was thinking it would be four and some change.

I got on that scale and the four never appeared. It was a digital scale, so it blinked a couple of times, and then it gave me the bad news: 510.

Oh shit! I weigh 500 pounds, I thought.

I remember Luscious Liz's reaction when she heard the number.

"Five hundred and ten pounds, oh my God, that doesn't even sound like weight," she said. "That sounds like a flight number."

To be honest, the number did and didn't phase me. I didn't have a big emotional reaction. I didn't need to camouflage it from listeners, or anything like that. Maybe it was just because I was in the moment, but I reacted to it as a potential for entertainment more than anything else. That was probably because my mindset wasn't just on my health. Actually, I think Will went into the challenge more concerned about my health than I was. My mission came more from thinking what all of this would do for the show.

"All right, Will, we're starting at 510 pounds," I said.

After that, we announced the rules of the challenge—Will would pay me $1000 for every pound I lost; and the money would be split between the two charities of our choice. Will chose A Place Called Home. I chose my organization, Ida's Son Foundation, which supports The Children's Hospital and various local charities.

That's where we started. Even though I'd never successfully dieted before, I wasn't worried that I wouldn't be able to lose the weight. That was a good thing because, once we kicked it off, I knew that I really had to do this. Will had all of L.A.'s eyes on me. When he called into the show each week to check on me, he had a message for listeners, "Yo, make sure that you all keep him in line."

Suddenly, it seemed like everyone in Los Angeles was my nutritionist. When I went to a restaurant, people came up to my table.

"What you doing in here, man?" they said.

"I'm about to order a salad," I said.

"Okay, alright," they said.

I couldn't even pull up to a drive-through.

People literally came up to my car.

"Oh no, man, you got to win that money for them kids."

So I tried to focus. I'll admit that I wasn't eating great all through the whole challenge. But I got to the gym. Mostly, I started eating right. I pulled back on what I was eating and had some Lean Cuisines. I drank more water and realized that the less I ate, the less I wanted. I was serious about it. I knew that I had to pull this off for charity, for the show, for Will, for me, for everything.

And it worked. The first week, I lost 18 pounds.

"You lost 18 pounds," Liz said, like she couldn't believe it.

I was more realistic.

"But Liz, I'm 18 pounds off of 510 pounds," I said. "That's water weight. I haven't even started on the fat yet."

Still, that was $18,000 for charity. And it felt good.

When Will checked in that week, he celebrated. I celebrated, too. From then on, Will kept checking in once a week. I kept losing more and more. Then, I started feeling better. I could feel it during my workouts. I could see the difference in the way my face was looking. I had always known that weight could kill me, just like how people who smoke cigarettes know that they could get lung cancer—but still smoke—I had been living in a lot of denial. And, finally, I wasn't in denial anymore. I was acknowledging that I had control over the role that food played in my life—that there was a direct relationship between how and what and when I ate with how much I weighed. For the first time, ever, my eating wasn't compulsive. I was in control of my eating and my weight. And it felt great.

Man, I can do this, I thought. *I'm starting a lifestyle. I'm losing this weight.*

And lose weight I did. I still have a picture of when I hit 399 pounds. I remember that day because you couldn't tell me that I wasn't thin. As far as I was concerned, I looked anorexic.

Overall, the weight loss challenge was very successful. We had decided that we would run the challenge until August, and on the final day, August 8, 2002, Will came into the studio for the grand finale. I had lost 111 pounds, and he presented me with a giant check for $111,000, which I still have at the house. It was a great show. Even better, I felt really good—in my body—and about myself.

When I got off the air at 10:00 am that day, as I always did, I left the station. Only, this day, I drove straight to this Mexican restaurant, La Fogata's, which made these nachos that I loved. I mean it was that direct, like I went there before I even checked to see if my house was on fire.

I didn't think much about the nachos. It was just a treat, then I'd get back into my new diet and lifestyle. During the weight loss challenge, my whole attitude towards food and my health had really changed. I finally felt that having a healthy lifestyle was something I could do. So, in my mind, I was still on the program.

But then, the next night, I stopped at Kentucky Fried Chicken. And it just went on from there. It was like I didn't even realize how out of control I was—until I was totally out of control. I didn't know how much weight I was putting on, but I could feel it creeping back, week—by week. Finally, when I did get back on the scale, it said I had gained 8 pounds. That hit me, but not hard enough. I kept eating. The next time I got on the scale, a month later, I had gained another 20 pounds. Just like that.

Oh, shit, man, this is coming back, I thought.

When I felt the weight coming back on, something changed for me. So many people in Los Angeles knew about the challenge and had been calling me out on my eating habits throughout it. But then, once I started putting the weight on, it was like nobody mentioned it anymore. I'm sure my crew saw it. There's no way they could have not seen it. I don't think I ever allowed them to feel comfortable enough to say something to me about it.

I stayed off the scale and tried to ignore what was happening for as long as I could. But it was impossible for me to deny how much my weight had gone down—and then up—when I got a new acting role, I was regularly seeing myself onscreen.

Right around the time of the weight loss challenge, I had been asked to play the part of Aquarius on the television show *Fastlane*. The show's creator, McG, is a hip hop head. I had already done a cameo in his *Charlie's Angels* film; so he had me in mind for the part from the beginning. He had come to the station, told me about Aquarius and asked if I wanted to play him. I liked McG. He's very animated and enthused; he made me feel comfortable. He was the perfect person for me to work with.

While we were working together, McG was great about being open to input on the show. Originally, my character was a drug dealer; but I told him that I didn't want to play a drug dealer. McG was down with that. We came to terms. He made Aquarius a hustler instead. Aquarius was cool with the streets. He was cool with the police. If a cat needed two front row seats to a concert, Aquarius could get that.

McG was the perfect guy to work with because you could get him on the phone—you could talk to him. When it got to a point where my wardrobe started looking crazy, I was like: "Dude, what do you have me wearing?"

"What's the problem?" he asked.

"They got me in dashikis and looking like a tarot card reader, or wearing slacks with dress shirts and shit."

"What do you want to wear?" he said. "Just tell me."

So I told him that no real hustlers dressed like that, and he ended up making it so that Aquarius wore normal stuff, like T-shirts and Sean John sweatsuits.

I loved doing the show. It wasn't like I ever thought I'd be a movie star or anything like that, because music and radio were my loves. But it was crazy to find myself sitting in my trailer, or trading lines with Bill Bellamy, Peter Facinelli and Tiffani Thiessen.

I used to go in so over-prepared. It was not like radio at all, because radio is my world. I can have fun. I can be loose. I can do this, do that, or whatever. But with TV, I didn't want them to call cut during a shot because I forgot a line, or because I didn't hit a mark. During that time, I would be out at the clubs on a Friday or Saturday night, sitting in the corner; and people would see me mouthing words. They probably thought I was crazy. But that was just me going over my lines for the next week's shoot.

Usually, I nailed my lines in one take. But, one night, we were shooting this scene, and I had some dialogue with Bill Bellamy and Peter Facinelli. I had to deliver it while we were walking. Then, I was supposed to jump in my car and drive off, so it had to be one smooth roll through the whole take. There was no chance to cut up two takes and edit them together. But I just could not get it. I must have had to do ten takes. Because we were shooting at night, it was so cold. I'd be walking back to my mark, and I'd see people in the crew with jackets and blankets on. I felt so badly. That didn't help matters any, though. I just could not nail it down. There were even a couple of takes where I got so far along that I had my hand on the door of the car. Still, I'd mess it up, and I'd have to go back and start again.

"I'm sorry," I said. "I'm sorry."

That was the most takes that I've done on anything that I've been on. The rest of the time it was always cool on the set.

Fastlane started off strong in the ratings. It was a fun show with great production values, and people really liked it. It hit for a while. I don't know why it didn't hit more. But then, it started getting moved around on the Fox schedule, and it got cut into by the baseball season. The next thing I knew, after the end of the first season, this guy came up to me at the grocery store one night.

"Hey, Big," he said and introduced himself as one of the show's producers.

We chatted for a bit and then he just laid it down.

"We're not coming back," he said.

That's how I found out we'd been canceled.

During *Fastlane's* run, which was one season from the fall of 2002 to the spring of 2003, the writers had written it into the show that Aquarius was losing weight, because it was so obvious from week to week. That felt pretty good. And then, after the challenge ended, I had to go into the studio to do some dubs for the show. So that basically involved me sitting there for a few hours, looking at what was on the screen and matching my voice to the words I had spoken in front of the camera. I was sitting there with my headphones on, listening to the playback, and watching the timer to see when I needed to speak. As soon as my character came onto the screen, I saw it.

Oh, fuck, I thought.

I could see my weight loss right there on the screen, and I knew I had gained a bunch of weight since then. It was so obvious to me. I looked real casually at my homeboy, Joe Grande, who was in the studio with me. He literally did a double take when he saw me on the screen. I could tell that he saw it, too.

Joe and I were talking as we walked out of the studio.

"Joe, man, I put some weight on," I said.

He didn't sugar coat it.

"Yeah, Big, when you came on that screen, I was like, 'Oh, wow.'"

26

BECAUSE I COULD

My career was golden. But my life was not. The more weight I gained back, the more I avoided the scale. I didn't want to see it. It was too hard to face the fact that I had taken off 111 pounds, but now, here I was, grabbing the old 8X shirt again. And the worst part was that I knew everybody else could see it, too. After the publicity the weight loss challenge garnered, and my stint on *Fastlane,* more people were aware of my weight—how much it had gone up and down, than ever before.

For the first time in my life, I became self-conscious about my weight. I felt badly about it and found myself kind of sucking in my gut around other people. I'd never done anything like that before. I mean I was Big Boy from the Morning Obsession billboards. I was fat. That was just who I was. Or who I'd been. Suddenly, I experienced feelings I'd never had in my entire life as Big Boy. I felt shame, embarrassment, and a sense of failure. I found myself conversing with myself, internally, about all of this in a way I'd never done before.

I'm sure a lot of you can relate to this. It's got to be the worst feeling in the word, that little voice that tells you that you're too fat, too dumb, too whatever, and that you'll never be happy because of it. Believe it or not, this was the first time I'd ever gone through these feelings. As fat as I'd always been, and even with some of the dumb shit that I got into when I was younger, I'd always felt good about myself. I guess it was all of that good love that my Mom had always given me. But as much as she'd loved me no matter how big I was, or what I did, she'd also always taught me to do my best. Now, I felt like I'd really let myself down. As anyone who's heard that little voice knows, the real problem is that once it starts up in your head, it can make you feel so badly about yourself that it's hard to do anything about it.

Suddenly, my weight wasn't just an issue of vanity. For the first time in my life, I started to feel the fat. Up until then, when I'd been at 500 pounds, I'd been doing the splits and exercising. I mean my trainer, Rod, he was an ex-Marine, and before the weight loss challenge, he'd have me running up a flight of twenty stairs like thirty-five or forty times in a row. He'd work me so hard I felt like I had to throw up. Instead of letting me slow down, he'd give me a trashcan and tell me to go ahead and get sick. He even used me as an incentive to get his other clients moving.

"Man, Big Boy does this," he told them. "You should be able to do it." Or "Big Boy at 500 pounds would run you guys into the ground."

Hell, I used to worry about my heart exploding during those workouts. But, other than that, my health was good. I never had high blood pressure, diabetes—none of that. It's not like my doctor didn't tell me to lose weight. Still, given that I weighed 500 pounds, I'd always been pretty fit.

Now that I had lost the weight, and then gone back up in size, something had changed. I noticed it when I was walking through the Bob Hope Airport in Burbank to catch a flight to Vegas. I had to stop and catch my breath. I had never had to do anything like that before. Around that time, I started to get this pinch in my back, where my leg would go numb. Sometimes I had shooting pains up and down my leg. I figured that I had a pinched nerve, so I went to see a chiropractor. Again, I'd never had anything like that before. For the first time, I started to feel like I was getting sleep apnea, which I'd also never had before. Sure, since I'd first gotten really big, I'd had to sleep sitting up, but because I was used to adapting to the ways that my size impacted my life, it was my norm. I'd never had any issues beyond that.

Just like that, there was this whole new ration of problems. I could've ignored them, and not paid attention to the signs, like I'd denied that my weight was a death sentence for my whole life. But I finally felt badly enough that I couldn't live in denial anymore. I knew everything was coming. Everything. And I knew it was going to come very fast because, just in the few months it had taken me to put the weight back on, so much had jumped on me.

Dude this isn't feeling good, I thought.

I didn't know what to do. I had lost weight. But it hadn't worked. And now, I really felt like there was no way I could diet and exercise my way to thin, or even to anything less than morbidly obese, especially not for a lifetime. So, instead of going back to eating less, like I had been for those six months of the weight loss challenge, I started eating more.

At first, I almost had this feeling like I had earned the right to eat as much as I wanted to eat and be as big as that meant I would be.

I got the money, and I can go buy that chicken, I thought.

I wasn't the poor kid who could only get a dollar from his Mom for a Big Mac as a special treat. I wasn't the homeless kid who had to eat whatever he could find in the mission kitchen. I was Big Boy. Like the rock star that could have all the booze, cocaine and groupies he wanted, I could have access to anything. Only, all I wanted was food. I had gained weight my whole life; now, my eating went to a whole new place.

I lived alone, and most people who live alone would probably go buy a small pizza. Not me. I bought the extra large pizza and ate the whole thing. Not in one sitting, but it'd be in the refrigerator, and I'd eat it over the course of a day. The next day, it started all over again. While I was at POWER, I spent all day thinking about what I was going to eat after work, even if we'd had a lunch meeting at a restaurant and I'd eaten a big, full meal. I literally watched the clock because I wanted to go to Kentucky Fried Chicken on my way home. I planned my day around meals. Then, on my way home from work, just like I'd promised myself, I stopped at Kentucky Fried Chicken and got the 14-piece or the 20-piece Family Feast. For myself. Of course, I probably weighed *more* than a family by this point; but I don't think it's supposed to work that way.

I love to cook, too. So I made these huge meals, telling myself I was cooking extra and saving some for leftovers. But really, I was cooking way more than a person that lived alone really needed. I might fry up a couple of packages of chicken wings and eat all of them during the course of a day. I'd make a pot of pasta with chicken and broccoli. I'd make a pot of soup. Then, as if that wasn't enough food, I'd go buy ten chicken wings and ten legs and throw them in, too. I'd stay at home by myself, watching movies and eating, on and off, for hours. Finally, it got to the point where something changed inside of me.

This isn't good, I thought. *This is getting excessive.*

There were times when I would wake up just to eat. There were times when I would eat and then go lay down. I can remember waking up choking because I had undigested food in my system. There I was, sitting in my TV room, eating myself to death. And I knew it. I wasn't diagnosed with anything that might have been considered a side effect of my weight—like high blood pressure or diabetes—but I knew everything was coming. I felt it.

I needed a change in my life, but I didn't know where to start. Then, I met two people who would change my life forever. The first was at a movie premiere in early 2003. This cat came up to me and shook my hand.

"Hey Big Boy," he said.

"Hey, man, what's up?" I said.

"You ever seen that movie *Varsity Blues?*" he asked.

"Yeah, sure," I said, not getting where he was going with this.

"Ron Lester, the big guy," he said.

"Yeah," I said, uncertainly.

Usually when someone came up and started saying something about a big guy, it was about how he'd had a heart attack or died. Maybe Ron Lester had died.

"It's me," he said. "I'm Ron Lester."

There was no way this was Ron Lester. This dude was skinny.

"No," I said.

So he handed me his card, and he really was Ron Lester.

I couldn't get over it. I just kept staring at his face. He looked like a completely different person.

"Man, what the fuck did you do?" I said.

"I had a gastric bypass surgery," he said.

After that, we exchanged phone numbers. I watched him go to his seat. I was sitting about ten rows behind him, crammed into an aisle seat, like I'd been doing at concerts and movies for years. As I watched, he slid along the row until he reached his seat, and then, he slid into it easily, just like anybody else. That made a big impression on me. But at that point, I wasn't even thinking about the procedure he'd gotten. I was just celebrating this guy's weight loss.

A few days later, I did call Ron to ask him more about what he'd done and how much weight he'd lost. He started telling me about how he had weighed 508 pounds when he went in for his surgery. I heard that. He had weighed 2 pounds less than me at the time that he had decided to do something about it.

And then he started describing how he'd flatlined on the table while they were operating on him. That pulled me back.

Oh, man, he flatlined, I thought. *Shit, I'm cool.*

But the more we talked about the surgery, the more I got how much it had changed his life. And it started to get inside of my mind.

I thought to myself: *Here I am, 33 years old, 500 pounds. Do I have more years behind me than I have in front of me? Well, you don't see too many 500-pound 66-year-old men walking around, do you? So the answer is YES!*

I didn't want to die. I started listening harder.

He told me that he'd had something called the duodenal switch, which I had never even heard of until then. I went online and started looking up the duodenal switch. I learned that it is the most extreme form of gastric bypass available, and that where he had gotten it done—the Advanced Obesity Center in Georgia—is considered one of the top centers in the country. I also looked at the so-called regular gastric bypass, which is a procedure called the Roux-en-Y, as well as another technique called the Fobi Pouch. There are a few different surgery options. I looked into them all.

I compared the weight loss results, and the percentage of people that put the weight back on after they'd had their procedure done. The duodenal switch was the most drastic. It was pretty much irreversible. Instead of shrinking the stomach, like the regular gastric bypass did, it actually involved doing a more complicated procedure to the digestive track. It also had the best results: patients lost the most weight and kept it off.

So, the duodenal switch was the procedure that kind of jumped out at me. I figured that I was in the most extreme weight category, so I probably needed the most extreme operation. It wasn't like I was planning to fail, but I'd seen people who'd lost weight from a gastric bypass surgery, only to put the weight right back on. And after what I'd been through following the weight loss challenge, I was honestly scared that I might yo-yo like that again. If I was going to do something, I wanted to make sure I got the biggest kick in the ass.

I spent probably the next eight months researching the procedure, reading about what was involved, going into online chat rooms and asking questions of people who'd gone through the surgery themselves.

I knew I had to do something. I knew that if I didn't, I was going to die. But that didn't make it any easier to actually make the choice and move forward with it. I never thought that I'd get really skinny, but I knew I'd lose enough weight for me to be healthy going forward. And that made me pause.

What's going to happen to Big Boy? I wondered. *What about when I joke about myself? What's going to happen with all that?*

It was an identity struggle. I had built a lot of equity in being obese as far as the name, the billboards, what I looked like, what I went to when I cracked the mic, what the listeners gravitated towards, and what the conversations with artists and fans started on. I was *Big Boy*.

During this time, I had so many what-if moments when I wondered if I could really do it. Sometimes it got pretty dark.

Would I be funny?

Would I be entertaining?

What would I talk about on the air?

It was all so unfamiliar to me. I'd been big my whole life. I'd been Big Boy on Power 106 for almost a decade by then. If I had the surgery, I'd be going into a land of the unknown. It was a gamble. I worried that if I wasn't big anymore, everything I had would go away. I finally talked to my producer Jason about it.

"Your size isn't who you are," he said.

Hearing that helped, but I still questioned it for many months before I could let my fears go. At the same time, I was still at war with myself about my eating and the weight I had gained. It got to the point where I kept having this thought: *Is that piece of chicken worth it? If it is, then fine, keep doing it. But you're going to die.*

And then something just came over me. It reminded me of my friend Chris McCrary, who'd always smoked. Then, one New Year's Eve, he took his last cigarette and he said he was going to quit because, if he didn't, cigarettes were going to kill him. That cat flipped that cigarette and that was the last cigarette he's had in more than twenty years. Something like that started to happen to me. This was another one of those moments in the book of life when God handed me a pen. There was a blank page right in front of me, and I had to start filling in that page. I knew that one page could dictate what's on the next page, in the next chapter, or how the book ends. So I decided to write my page and change my life. First, I had to save my life.

27

THREE THINGS I NEVER, EVER DO

Before I had the chance to make a decision about getting gastric bypass surgery, I had a second life-changing meeting. It happened on a Saturday night in Las Vegas in April of 2003. I was there for a promo weekend with the POWER listeners. It was a standard trip, except that I had to do a club that night, and I never do appearances when I go to Vegas. But DJ E-Man from *The Neighborhood* and I had to appear at a club; and that's just how it was. The club had sent me transportation, but they only sent over one car. There were probably ten or fifteen cats in my crew. Not everybody would fit.

"You guys go first," I said. "Then they'll have to come back and pick me up."

That's how we got over to the club. We did the same thing after I was done. By the time I got back to the Hard Rock Hotel where I had a room, I was done for the night.

I was walking through the casino to get to the elevator, when a beautiful woman with lovely, long hair stopped me.

"Hey, Big, it's Veronica," she said. "I called you today. My friend Erica gave me your number."

"I don't know why Erica gave you my number," I said. "I erased the message."

I wasn't unfriendly about it. But no one—and I mean no one—had my phone number. I wasn't trying to talk to anybody. So I couldn't understand how she had gotten my number like that. When I'd heard the message, I'd just deleted it. Being in the public eye, I've always had to be careful about my private life, just like how I watched out for my cats in the Pharcyde when I was keeping them safe on the road.

Now that Veronica was standing in front of me, though, I remembered having met her once before at the Wiltern Theater with her friend Erica. I did know Erica well enough for her to have my number. I'd gotten her some tickets for a Jay-Z show at the Wiltern. That night, Erica had come up to say thank you and introduced me to Veronica, along with several other girlfriends. I didn't think anything of it because I didn't usually trip off meeting women. I couldn't help just watching them as they walked away because they had some nice asses. (Truth must be told). But that was it.

Now that we were talking, Veronica seemed nice, so we sat down. She was with her friend Jennifer. I was with Tattoo, Ray and Louie.

Veronica told me that she and Jennifer were in Vegas with Jennifer's cousin, who had taken off on them with their money, IDs, and the keys to where they were staying. She didn't know what to do because she had no way of getting back to her place. Then, before I knew it, I guess we were kind of flirting. I was clowning about my weight, and she got right in there with me.

"You've got a beautiful body," she said.

So we started playing opposites.

"Your toes are nasty," I said.

"No, they're not," she said. "I know I have cute feet."

I gave her a playful look like she was crazy.

"You have nasty feet," I said. "Ray, get over here and see this girl's feet."

Ray came over. I introduced him to Veronica and Jennifer.

"Look at how nasty her feet are," I said.

"Yeah, you have some busted feet," Ray said.

"No, I don't," Veronica said. "I don't care what you tell me. I have nice feet."

We talked some more. Finally, I decided to play nice. She really did have beautiful toes.

"I'm just kidding," I said.

We hung out a little bit more, and I could feel that there was just something about her. Finally, it was time for her to leave, and for me to head to the airport to catch my flight home to Los Angeles. But I didn't want to leave Veronica stranded.

"I want to make sure you guys get home okay," I said. "I know that Jennifer's cousin left you."

And then, as we were all getting ready to leave, I did three things that I never, ever do:

I gave her my real name, Kurt, which I never give.

I gave her my real phone number.

I let her use my restroom. No one uses my restroom.

I never let listeners, or anybody else, into my hotel room when I'm out on the road for work. Never. I dropped so many guards that night.

I even mentioned it to Ray.

"Damn, dude, I just gave this girl my real name," I said.

Then, we went downstairs. We were just talking and talking the whole time. I got a cab, which her friends and I shared. I jumped out at Southwest to fly home and had the taxi drop them off at where they were staying. After that, I found myself thinking about Veronica and wanting to make sure she got home safe. So I called.

"Did you guys get home okay?" I asked.

After that, we started talking on the phone. It wasn't ever like I wanted to get her or I was making a big play for her. She was just really nice, I enjoyed her conversation. We could just talk and talk. Normally, I'm the type of person who doesn't really like being on the phone with people. Because I lived alone at the time, I could control how much conversation I had with people, and I was cool with that. But with Veronica, I noticed that I enjoyed talking with her on the phone more and more. It was always good conversation. I liked that she wasn't just talking about what we did on air that day. I don't mind talking to people about the show. But I liked that she wasn't on some Big Boy trip. She knew what I did, but she wasn't a listener. She wasn't asking me to give a shout out to her brother or whatever. With Veronica, I knew she was calling to talk to Kurt, not Big Boy. It got to the point where we talked every day, and we literally fell asleep on the phone together.

If anything, I didn't think she was ready for how sedated me and my crew really were. Like, we'd get on my bus, and there'd be no smoking, no drinking, no girls; and the music we would play while we're driving would be something mellow. She was probably like, *These guys suck.* But I knew I didn't have to impress her.

It got to a point where, when I saw her phone number on my caller ID, I'd make sure that I could take her call and talk to her for a good, long time. And then, I wanted to see her more and more. We'd be talking and I'd throw something out to her.

"I'm going to be at this club on Friday night," I said. "Why don't you come out?"

So after we'd been talking for a few weeks, we started hanging out as more of a group thing with my crew and her friends. And then, it took off from there. One night, after we were all hanging out, I brought it up to Ray after she went home.

"I'm going to get her," I said.

"Nah," Ray said.

"I bet you I'm going to get her," I said.

We shook on it and that was that.

I wasn't looking for a relationship at the time. Like I said, I didn't have a problem getting girls because I was always a guy that people wanted to be around. I was funny. Of course, when I became Big Boy at POWER106, I knew that there were women who wanted to get with me because of my name. But I was never into that. I'd had a girlfriend for seven years, and when that ended about six months before meeting Veronica, I'd kept to myself.

I was like, *I'm cool on my own.*

Maybe I was self-conscious about my weight. I mean, let's be honest, I'm pretty sure there were a lot more women who didn't mess with me because of my size. However, no one ever told me to my face that she wasn't interested because she didn't like fat guys. But that's why it was so great with Veronica. Because we started out as friends, and we just really enjoyed each other's conversation, I never worried about it.

After a few weeks of always seeing each other in a big group, Veronica started coming over to my house, just one-on-one. Again, it felt more like friends than a super serious dating situation. I think that's what made it so great. We played my favorite game, Scattergories, watched TV, and just hung out. Then, one day, we kissed; and that was it.

I never felt weird about eating around Veronica or like I had to eat less in front of her than I did when I was alone—although I probably did, just because we were having such a good time doing other things. I sometimes thought that Veronica's friends were wondering what she was doing, going for me—or that she was asking herself why she was falling for this fat ass. I never mentioned it to her, though. I just let myself feel glad that she seemed to be falling for me like she was.

28

AS SOON AS I WAKE UP,
I'LL HAVE A NEW LIFE

The whole time that I was getting to know Veronica, I was doing research about the different weight loss surgeries. My running into Ron Lester had made a big impression on me. And I knew it was time for me to finally do something about my weight or face the fact that I might die. And soon.

After looking into everything, I decided that the duodenal switch, which Ron had undergone, was also the best for me. I started consulting Ron's doctor about getting everything in order for me to get it done.

At this point, Veronica and I had been dating for about four months, I knew I had to talk to her about it. One night, when we were lying in bed, and the room was really dark, I just started talking. I didn't tell her how badly I'd been feeling because I didn't want to worry or upset her, but I tried to be honest otherwise.

"Baby, I need to talk to you about something," I said.

"What is it, baby?" she asked.

"I've been doing research and I'm thinking of getting gastric bypass surgery," I said.

"Baby don't," she said.

"I really need to do something about my weight," I said.

"Okay, but why the surgery?" she said. "Why not just lose weight? Why not just eat right, and work out and do it that way?"

"I've tried that," I said. "And you know, I've done research on the surgery. And my friend Ron Lester got it. And I really think it's what I need to do. I feel like I've got more years behind me than in front of me if I don't."

Veronica ended up supporting my decision. But it almost made me feel good that she hadn't wanted me to get the surgery at first. That meant I didn't have to worry that she secretly wanted me to lose weight or be some skinny dude.

Soon after our conversation, I started making plans to go to Georgia to have the procedure done. Normally, people go through six to eighteen months of preparation that includes a major psychological evaluation. But Ron Lester got things rolling by calling his doctor, who ended up doing my surgery, too—and after this doctor and I had only been in talks for a few weeks, he called me.

"I've got a slot available," my doctor said. "Can you be here in two weeks?"

"I can do that," I said.

"Lose as much weight as you can safely and get here," he said. "You'll be here for ten days."

I essentially got bumped to the front of the line because of my fame, which meant that I was able to have my surgery done in November 2003. I had some time off coming at the end of the year, so I made arrangements to fly to Georgia then. I didn't want my family there because I knew that they would worry too much. And I didn't want to put this on Veronica either, since we'd only been dating for a few months. I told her I wanted to go alone.

"That's just crazy," she said. "You have to have somebody there with you."

I still wasn't into that idea. I've always been someone who's taken care of things on his own. At the same time, it was hitting me how serious my feelings for Veronica were becoming. Around this time, I had a thought about Veronica that was just crazy, *Damn, dude, she reminds me of my Mom.* People know how I feel about my Mom, and I'd never compared anyone to her. This was serious. I realized what would make me really happy.

"When I wake up from surgery, I want you to be the first person I see," I said to Veronica.

She was relieved that I was going to let her be there with me. She agreed.

I flew to the Advanced Obesity Surgery Center in Marietta, Georgia two days before my procedure, which was scheduled for November 28, 2003. As far as before and after photos go, I actually have some video footage of myself that was taken on the day I left for Georgia. My foundation does a turkey giveaway every year, so we were doing that for my Thanksgiving show. I ended up being on the local news that day. I had to go to the airport from there. I can't even tell you how crazy it is when I look back at that, especially given what came next.

When I arrived in Georgia, I went through several days of tests and preparations, including a physical exam and a stress test. Now, remember that the doctor had said that I should lose as much weight as I could. I had done my best. But when I got on the scale the night before my surgery, I was 510 pounds, just like I had been when I started my weight loss challenge with Will Smith. That meant I must have been even bigger than I'd thought going into the surgery—probably 520 or 530 pounds, easy.

My doctor noticed my reaction to my weight.

"You'll never weigh that again," he said.

I still wasn't so sure, not after the weight loss yo-yo I'd just been on.

Damn, how does he know? I wondered.

The next morning, I had to be over to the Center for my surgery around five in the morning. I woke up early in my hotel room, got ready, grabbed my bags, and jumped in a cab. When I arrived, the attendant put me in this little waiting area. I was in there by myself, watching the news. It was so quiet that it felt like I was the only patient at the hospital. Then, a nurse came in and handed me a gown.

"Put this on," she said. "They're going to take you to surgery soon."

I got changed, put my belongings into a bag they had given me and waited for them to come and get me. Another nurse entered the room.

"Alexander," he said.

"Yes," I said.

"We're ready for you," he said. "Do you need any help?"

"No, I got it."

It wasn't exactly graceful, but I got my 500 pound self up onto the gurney he had waiting for me. As I lay there, they rolled me into the operating room. I had been calm up until then, but that's when it got real. And I don't mean surreal, either. I mean like so fucking real.

Oh shit, this is happening, I thought.

I wasn't having second thoughts. I couldn't believe that all of the conversations, and online research and travel had all ended here. They moved me onto the surgical table. I looked around. The operating room seemed gigantic from where I was lying, even with the little bit I could see by turning my head. I was lying under these lights. They looked huge.

They strapped my arms down.

"Mr. Alexander, how are you feeling?" a man asked.

He was holding a mask in his hand. He introduced himself to me as my anesthesiologist.

"I'm going to put this on you," he said.

He put the rubber mask over my face. Now it was realer than real.

"Count down from 10," he said.

"Ten . . . nine . . . eight . . . ," I said.

I knew there was a risk, that something like three percent of gastric bypass patients didn't make it through surgery. Of course, anytime there's a statistic like that, your mind goes right for it. But I wasn't afraid of dying. I knew I was going to die anyway if I didn't do something about my weight. I figured that I'd rather die trying to do something about it and give myself the chance to finally have a better life.

God, just wake me up, I thought. *As soon as I wake up, I'll have a new life.*

The next thing I knew, someone was speaking to me.

"Mr. Alexander, you're done," he said. "You're done."

I just lay there, slowly coming back to consciousness.

Finally, I opened my eyes and rolled them over to the side of the bed. Sure enough, Veronica was walking up. She was the first person I saw, just like I'd asked her to be. It was like she was my angel. I could feel that I had a tube in my nose. I tried to point at the tube. Finally, they pulled it out for me. As they cleaned me up from the surgery, I could feel all of this blood coming into my ears. But I was alive.

Dude, I made it, I thought.

It was a laparoscopic procedure, which meant they only made six small incisions in my stomach and did the surgery using these small knives on wires. Later, on the same day of the surgery, I was already sitting up in my bed; but I still had to stay in the hospital for three days to recover. Veronica was there the whole time. She took such good care of me. In the first hours after the surgery, she sat by my bed and fed me broth, which was all I could eat at that point.

After a few days, I was back up and around again, back in my rental car and back at my hotel. I had to stay out in Atlanta for another six days after the surgery because they had to put a tube in me and make sure I was well enough for them to clear me to travel back to Los Angeles. During this time, Veronica flew back to L.A. ahead of me. I had a portable studio with me so that I could broadcast from the hotel because I never wanted to be off the air for too long. Overall, I think I only missed my show for three days during that whole procedure.

Everything had gone smoothly; and finally, they cleared me to fly home. Ten days after I'd had the procedure, I turned in my rental car, got on a plane, and flew back to Los Angeles. I was already 30 pounds lighter. I felt amazing. I remember bouncing through the airport, feeling so light and full of life and energy.

As soon I got home, I got myself into a routine. Because my procedure purposely caused me to experience malabsorption—which meant that my body wasn't absorbing fat in the way that a normal person would—it was very important for me to make sure that I was getting enough calories and nutrients. Anything that was fat and greasy, I'd malabsorb that; the procedure would kick the bad stuff out of my system. But it's not like I just went and sought out the bad stuff. It threw everything out of my system—the good stuff too. So I had vitamins I needed to take and a whole regimen during the day. At first, I was only allowed to have liquids. Then, I introduced myself to soft food again. In a couple of weeks, I could eat some of the things I wanted. It was great. I was eating food that I loved *and* losing weight.

I was going through clothes like it was ridiculous. I'd buy something thinking this was my new size; in two weeks, it was gone. I was losing weight so fast that I couldn't hold a wardrobe.

I was celebrating it, but at the same moment, it felt crazy. First, I got down to like 400 pounds. You couldn't tell me I didn't look immaculate. I looked so different. When I cracked 350 pounds, I couldn't believe how skinny I looked, not knowing that I was still going to lose another hundred.

It was the same thing with sizes. When I went from an 8X shirt into a 5X shirt, I was modeling because I felt like I looked so good. Going from a size 68 pants to a size 60 was crazy. Then, I started cracking into the 50s. I remember that when I hit a size 52 pants, I just couldn't believe it.

Size 52, are you serious?

People measure their weight loss accomplishments in all different ways. For me, it was all about the seatbelt extension. The first time I flew and buckled my seatbelt without needing an extension, that was so monumental for me—not to mention opening the tray table over my lap. Going to Footlocker and buying an outfit—I'd never gone into Footlocker and bought an outfit for myself before. As far as I was concerned, that damn outfit might as well have been an Armani suit. This was a whole new life, and I was looking good.

29

GRINDING DOWN

Everything after my gastric bypass surgery was good. And then, a couple of months in, something changed. I started to grind down. I had a bad taste in my mouth. I was dizzy and lightheaded. Sometimes, I had no choice but to just go lay down, no matter what I was doing. My fingers would lock up. I'd feel the worst pain in them. I had to start taking all of my showers on my knees because, if the water was too hot, I'd black out. If I fell in the shower, I'd get banged up. Sometimes I'd black out in the shower anyhow. If I was on my knees, at least I didn't have far to fall. One night, I was at a George Lopez concert. I started laughing and blacked out.

I didn't want my family to worry, so I was trying to keep things positive and light for them. But one day, they were all over at the house. I was trying to keep up with the conversation and the fun we were all having, and I just couldn't do it. I pulled Veronica aside and told her what was going on. I needed her to tell my family that I was sorry but they had to go because I couldn't hang out right then.

As soon as they were gone, I lay down. I was so cold, and nothing that I did seemed to warm me up. Finally, I had like four or five blankets on me. Even then, I was still cold.

Another time, I came home, and as soon as I walked in and said hello to Veronica, it was almost like I started having a seizure. I didn't really know what was going on, but Veronica told me later on how scared she was because my eyes rolled to the back of my head. I was lying there on the floor, gasping for air.

"I'm going to call an ambulance," Veronica said.

"No, they can't come," I said. "They can't see that it's Big Boy from POWER 106."

Terrified as she was, she respected my wishes. Ten or fifteen minutes later, it passed. We had no idea what had just happened. All we could figure out was that my proteins were low, so I stayed down there on the floor. She fed me a protein drink through a straw. Finally, I felt okay again—not great, but at least okay.

The one upside to all of this was that Veronica and I were closer than ever. We never really talked about our relationship or put a label on it. But when I first got sick, she called in to her job one day to tell them that she needed to stay home and help me. Later that day I overheard her on the phone with one of her girlfriends, describing how it had all gone down:

"I just told them my man is sick," she said.

GASP, she said her man, I thought.

I called my boy Ray.

"Hey remember that dollar we bet?" I said. "Bring it over. I got her. She said 'Her Man.' I think I'm her boyfriend now."

My life could not have been better, but I had never felt worse. And I had no idea why. I called my doctor and told him about my symptoms. He kept telling me to take more proteins. Or more vitamins. Or more liquids. Every time he had a solution, I'd get hopeful. But nothing was helping. I'd be real careful about my proteins, just like he said to be, then I'd still feel the same: bad.

Finally, before I had even lost my first 100 pounds, I had to fly back to Georgia for some tests.

I sat in my doctor's office, just wanting him to make me feel better.

"Something's going on," I said.

He gave me a blank look that scared me. Here he was, the guy that I had put all of my faith in, and he was looking at me like he didn't know what to tell me. So I flew back to Los Angeles without any more answers than I'd had before my trip.

Like I had done before deciding to have the surgery, I went online and started reading and posting in forums dedicated to gastric bypass. I looked for other people like me who were blacking out, losing their thoughts, having a bad taste in their mouth. But no one was going through anything like I was. They all felt fine.

No one could tell me anything, but I knew something was wrong. I flew back to Georgia again within the next month.

"What's going on?" I asked. "This is not normal."

My doctor did more tests. I just hoped that this time he'd find something.

"We don't see anything that's abnormal," he said.

So I went home to Los Angeles again. For the next few months, I went back to Georgia several more times, just trying to get some information that could help me. But my doctor still didn't know anything about what was happening to me. All I could do was keep taking my protein and my vitamins. Because the duodenal switch was kicking them out of my body just as fast as I could take them, I was ingesting them regularly, all day, and all night. For most people who had gone through the same procedure, this was enough. But me, I started dwindling down. There were times I felt so bad that I would just lie down on the floor and I couldn't get up. Veronica would take a straw and put the protein in my mouth and feed it to me that way.

It didn't help that I couldn't sleep through the night. With the duodenal switch, I was always purging stuff out of my system, which meant I was always in the bathroom. I could never get a good, full night's sleep. It got that I was so tired and weak that I had to lie down all of the time. I couldn't get off the bed. I couldn't get off the floor. I couldn't do anything. Even lying down was bad for me, though, because those were times I should have been up taking proteins and vitamins. Missing my proteins and vitamins just made me feel worse.

I was losing too much weight. I got so behind the curve that I couldn't catch up. I was in and out of the hospital. But no one could tell me what was wrong. I was trying to find a specialist; no one seemed to know anything. Sometimes it got really dark.

What the fuck did I do to myself? I thought.

Everything would have been different if I had gotten one of the bands or rings that they had at the time because those can be tightened and loosened. So if I'd started having any kind of side effects, they could have just taken it right out of me, and I would have been fine. Of course, that's why I hadn't gotten a band or ring because I didn't trust myself not to loosen it myself by overeating. I had purposely gotten the most extreme procedure. Now, I was dealing with the most extreme consequences.

Sometimes I wondered if I was dying. That's how badly it felt. And the worst part was, because no one knew what was wrong with me, no one knew how to make me better. There seemed to be no end in sight. I could never tell myself that things would be better in the morning. For all I knew, they would be worse. And they did get worse before they got better. It was bad. Really bad.

There was no hiding the fact that something was going on with me, either. Right after the surgery, people came up to me all of the time to congratulate me on how good I looked. Now, they were coming up to me to express concern.

"You need to stop losing weight."

"Are you gonna stop?"

"What are you trying to get down to?"

It wasn't just how skinny I was, either. I looked sick. The whites of my eyes were discolored to this yellowish shade, like I had jaundice. I always had bags under them. To this day, my wife can't look at pictures of me from that time because of how bad I looked, and all of the memories it brings back of how sick I was.

As sick as I was, and as horrible as I looked, I was not about to let it affect *Big Boy's Neighborhood*. Veronica tried to get me to call in sick to work so many times.

"Baby, they'll understand," she said. "If you tell them you're sick, it's okay."

"I've got to go in," I said.

On some mornings, though, I felt so bad that I had to call Jason.

"I don't think I can make it in today," I said.

"Okay," he said.

But I still didn't want to stay home. It felt like I was giving up on myself.

"No, you know what," I said. "If I get in the shower, I'll be able to pull it off."

And I did exactly that and made it into the station—just like I'd promised.

It wasn't just that I was worried about my spot at the top. Getting myself to work was like a small triumph. Plus, being on the air was therapeutic for me—just like it had been after Mom died. I ended up getting up and going to work every day. But it was a fight. I was constantly dehydrated. Sometimes I came into the station dragging an IV I'd been given for my fluids. Sometimes I'd be listening to my crew talk and I'd want to say something, but I couldn't find the words. It was like I was in a coma or something.

When I was on air, I constantly forgot what I was saying. Our producer, Jason, could always tell days when it was really bad. He always prepped me going into the day's show about what we were going to cover in the next few hours.

"Big, we're gonna talk about Mariah Carey's album debut," he said.

"Okay, cool," I said.

Ten seconds later, I went live on the air.

"POWER 106, Big Boy in the Neighborhood," I said.

I did the whole breakdown, turned my mic off, and swiveled around to look at Jason. He stood there, just looking at me, with this strange expression on his face.

"Everything cool?" I said.

I didn't realize that I hadn't said anything about what he'd just told me to talk about. I had totally forgotten the topic, and the fact that he'd cued me.

That's when Jason knew: *Oh, no, Big's not having a good day.*

I was trying so hard to hold it together. I'd be talking to a member of my crew, and when I tried to concentrate on his face, I'd pass out. I can't explain it exactly. I'd just be there, then I'd be gone. Sometimes I blacked out while I was on the air. When I got to the end of the show, I couldn't remember how it had gone. When I took off my headphones and pushed away from the console, I had to ask my crew how the show had all gone down.

"How was that?" I would ask.

"You made it through, you made it through," they would reassure me.

One day while I was on air, Jason walked over to this board we have in the studio where he writes the schedule and things we need to cover each day. He pointed at something, as if to say, "You need to read this." While he was pointing, I tried to focus in on the words. But I felt myself just fading out. Luckily, I was able to wrap up the break—"POWER 106 Big Boy"—which was the all clear. Then, I managed to turn the mics down, so the listeners couldn't hear what was going on in the studio. Then, I was out. Next thing I knew, I could feel Fuzzy pulling my pants up. My head was bleeding. I had fainted on the air, fallen, banged my head, and landed on the ground with my ass up. That was the worst incident to happen during that time, but it wasn't all that unusual. I was in and out of it every day.

Sometimes I couldn't sit up. So I'd lie on the floor while we did our show. Jason balanced the microphone near my mouth; I could talk without sitting up. One day, one of my partners, a brother named Minister Tony, came in and saw me lying on the floor, doing my show like that. It wasn't until then that he really got how bad it was for me. I had no strength to sit up.

"Brother, you alright?" he asked.

I didn't answer. Clearly, I wasn't.

I couldn't schedule anything in advance because I never knew how I'd feel when the time rolled around for the commitment. In the morning, we could set a late lunch meeting at 2:00 pm, that was fine because I was feeling okay. But, then, later that day, or even in the next moment, I felt like I'd been hit by a Mack truck. I couldn't sit up, talk, or think. So I certainly couldn't make it to a meeting. The worst part was that I never knew what I would feel like at the next moment. It was so bad, I couldn't even begin to describe the feeling. I just felt horrible, like the absolute worst. I tried never to cancel on a guest. But sometimes we had to because there was just no other choice. It'd be time to do the interview, and I couldn't talk or even hold my head up.

Sometimes I'd say my goodbyes, leave the station, and go out to my car, ready to drive home. The next thing I knew, Fuzzy was knocking on my car window.

"Big, you okay?" he said.

Without even realizing it, I'd been sitting there in my car for three hours. I did not know where I was or what I had been doing. Sometimes, I blacked out on the road while I was driving. Although I wasn't driving that much, because I was at home more, and friends including Fuzzy often offered to drive me places, I always thought that I could make it. I always did; but I can see now what a dangerous gamble I was taking. Thank God I didn't kill someone.

Again, this wasn't an occasional thing. This was every day. Every day I was blacking out. Every day I was fainting. Every day I was down on the floor. My body was just totally grinding down.

It was the least of my worries at the time, given everything else, but I looked crazy, too. My face looked sick. And my body—well, it was just nuts. I had lost so much weight, so quickly—I lost 150 pounds during the first year after my surgery—that I had big folds of excess skin hanging off of me. If I had been feeling better, I probably could have tightened up some at the gym. But with how badly I was doing, I couldn't exercise. I couldn't even pick up a ten-pound weight. Veronica and I went on a trip during this time, and I was struggling with the suitcases. When we got to the airport, the guy from Sky Cab picked up each suitcase with one hand and just started throwing them onto the conveyer belt. Another time, I was playing with Veronica, just playfully trying to hold her still, and she pushed me across the house. I was sliding across the floor on my socks because I couldn't even hold my ground against her.

Oh shit, I thought. *This is not good.*

30

HERE COMES MY STROKE

Month by month, my health kept getting worse. Then, that March 2004, it was time for the Los Angeles Marathon, which I had said I would do ten miles of for charity. Veronica tried to talk me out of it. I had no illusions that it was going to be anything other than rough. But my friend, Frankie, had just lost his battle with cancer at age 13. I wanted to take part in the marathon to raise money for The Children's Hospital in his honor.

"You're crazy," Veronica said. "Why would you say you'll do ten miles, knowing how you feel?"

"I made a promise to do ten miles for Frankie," I said. "I'm going to do it."

And I did.

I didn't run the race. That wasn't happening. But I walked the whole ten miles that I had said I would do. Even though it took me nearly eight hours, I made it to the end. When I got home, though, I was just done. I walked in the front door and fell to the ground. I had another one of those episodes where my eyes rolled back, and it was like I had to spit but nothing was coming out. I was lying on the floor, and Veronica was holding my hand.

"Baby, I'm going to call the ambulance," she said.

"No, I don't want you to call," I said.

"Well, I'm going to call your brother," she said. "I'm going to call your family."

"No, don't call anybody," I said.

I didn't want to worry anyone. I think a part of me didn't want to admit just how bad things really were.

My body was all kinds of messed up. I stopped losing weight, but it wasn't a good thing. It was because I had started getting so sick that I was gaining the wrong kind of weight. When I got on the scale late on a Wednesday, I weighed 240 pounds. By Friday morning, I weighed 297 pounds. That's how swollen I was. My ankles were so big, they were hanging over my shoes. Normally I wear shorts—I always have—but I couldn't anymore because they were so tight. Fuzzy or someone else was always asking me if I was okay. I had indentations in my ankles where my socks touched the skin. When I slid my finger in between my sock and my leg, even the gentlest touch of my finger left a mark. My body was just done.

I went to my primary doctor. He didn't know what it was. He told me to stop eating salt. I knew that wasn't it. I went to a herbologist. Nobody knew anything. And the scariest part was, from day to day, I never knew what was going to happen to me next.

Finally, my primary care doctor brought up a specialist named Dr. Quilici that he had first mentioned to me six months earlier. Quilici specialized in gastric bypass. My primary care doctor felt like he might be able to help. I was ready to try anything. But I wasn't exactly optimistic by this point, since no one else had been able to do anything for me. Still, I made an appointment and went into Dr. Quilici's office.

After Dr. Quilici examined me and ran some initial tests, he sat down with me to talk about his findings. Right away, he said something that floored me.

"I know what this is," he said.

I didn't entirely believe him since no one else had known. How could he be any different? But even just for him to say it out loud felt like a miracle.

Thank you, Jesus, I thought. I really felt like my prayers had been answered.

"What's happening here is your body is not grabbing enough protein and vitamins from what you eat," he said. "So it's releasing fluids out."

He started asking me about my symptoms. Every symptom matched his diagnosis. Just like that, after everything I'd been through, I had real information.

"When you first got your gastric bypass," he said, "you never caught up with your levels. Your body has constantly been trying to chase something that there was no way you could possibly catch."

"What can we do?" I asked.

"For one, you are losing weight," he said. "Let's try to keep you from doing that. But this is where you are right now. They say the odds of this happening are one thousand to one. You're that one."

"So what can we do?" I asked again.

"My friend, this is going to take months," he said. "I can't give you a pill and make this go away."

During that time, Dr. Quilici worked around my schedule. He admitted me to the hospital on my days off and gave me a bunch of tests.

While I was in the hospital for the first time, a doctor and a nurse walked into my room one day and looked at me in bed.

"How are you doing?" they asked.

Then they walked out. When they walked back in, they grabbed my chart.

"Okay, Alexander, Kurt, let me see your bracelet," the doctor said.

They both looked closely at my bracelet. I couldn't figure out what was going on. The doctor finally explained. When he had first looked at my test results, my levels were so low that he was expecting to walk in and see somebody much older than me—someone who was possibly on his deathbed. It didn't add up that I could be as young and otherwise healthy as I was with the levels that I had. No kidding.

"You need to be monitored," he said.

It was such a relief to be told that I actually had the chance to start feeling better soon. But I was that one in a thousand patient. I still couldn't find anyone else that was going through what I was going through. Then, the local news did a story on a lady who had undergone a procedure that was similar to mine, she couldn't stop losing weight either. Someone who worked at POWER with me came in the day after the story ran and started talking to me about it.

"Hey, are you gonna stop losing weight?" he asked.

"I don't know," I said.

"There's this lady on TV," he said.

"I know," I said. "I've been watching her too. I've been wanting to talk to her."

Then, just like that, the lady died. That did not make me feel optimistic.

A little while after that, I went into this store called Bell Sales, which is where I used to buy all of my fat clothes because they carried up to a size 10X. Obviously, I wasn't shopping for fat clothes anymore. When I walked in, the security officer recognized me because I had always shopped there. He must have seen that I wasn't looking good.

"Big Boy," he said. "You're still losing weight?"

"Yeah," I said.

"Can you stop?" he asked.

"I don't know," I said.

He got this look of concern on his face. And I couldn't blame him, given how I felt—and how badly I knew I looked.

"Man, there's a lady that's shopping here," he said. "She had the surgery. She can't stop losing weight either."

"Really?" I said.

It was the first time I'd felt hopeful in a long time.

"Yeah, she's having complications," he said. "Do you want to meet her?"

She was in the women's section that day, buying extra small sweat suits for herself. The security officer walked her over to me. When she turned around to face me, she looked dead. If I had seen this lady without knowing her story, I would have thought that she was dying from cancer or HIV, or that she had an extremely bad drug habit. As I stared at her, there was nothing reassuring to me about our meeting, because she had undergone the procedure before me. It made me worry that I was looking at what was down the road for me.

"Do you get lightheaded?" I asked her.

"Yeah, I get lightheaded."

"Do you black out?"

"Yeah."

"Do you get a bad taste in your mouth?"

"Yeah."

"What about your fingers? Do your fingers cramp up?"

"Yeah."

I wanted her to say no to something, but everything I was going through, she'd been through too. And then, it got worse.

"I had a heart attack," she said. "And then, I had a stroke. And when I woke up from the stroke, I had this accent."

I had noticed her accent while we were talking and thought she was from Germany. No, that was from the stroke. She was born in New Jersey and lived in Lancaster, just outside of Los Angeles.

"I'm not holding my vitamins and minerals," she said.

"I'm not holding mine either," I said.

"I was losing so much weight that they had to put this feeding tube in my chest," she said, showing it to me. "I have to wear a back-pack and it's got to pump all of these fluids and proteins into me."

"Nah, that hasn't happened to me," I said.

Yet, I thought. *Fuck, here comes my stroke. Here comes my German accent.*

The woman introduced me to her husband. We all talked for a few more minutes. Before I left, they gave me their number. I ended up leaving the store in a daze, without even shopping for anything because I was so torn up from hearing what this lady had gone through. I picked up my phone on the way to my car and called Veronica.

"Hey, I just met this lady," I said.

I told Veronica all about it, about how I was scared because everything that was happening to me had happened to her. How could I not assume that I was due for a heart attack and a feeding tube in my chest sometime soon, too?

"You need to listen to her," Veronica said. "Because everything that you're feeling, she's describing. You need to pay attention because you don't want that to be you."

I took the woman's number home and put it on my nightstand where I wouldn't lose it. I definitely wanted to talk to her some more. In the meantime, I was really freaked out, so I went and got more tests done. At least I was now working with Dr. Quilici, who seemed to have more of an idea of what was going on with me than anyone else had. But he had some scary news for me, too.

"You've got to be careful," he said. "You could send your heart into shock."

Of course, I thought of the lady and her heart attack.

"Your levels are getting low, and you could have a stroke," he said. That lady had a stroke, too.

"You're losing too much weight," he said. "This has got to stop."

"I can't stop it," I said. "I've tried."

"You're depleting," he said. "You could die."

Here was a doctor that didn't have a panic switch. I knew those were real words because everything else he had said to me had been the truth. He had told me that I needed to take my vitamin A, or I might go blind. That was right on. I hadn't been as good with my vitamin A as I should be. I had been losing my eyesight.

Finally, during one of my visits, Dr. Quilici came in and broke it down for me.

"You're not holding any of your vitamins," he said. "You're not holding *anything*. We're going to have to put a feeding tube in your chest."

"Okay," I said, trying to stay calm.

"Can you go into the hospital for two or three months?" he asked.

"No way, man," I said.

Not with my gig. We have a saying in radio: Here today, gone today.

If I had to be off the air for even two weeks, I'd be in trouble. Even when I went on vacation, I recorded bits in advance and left my crew behind to keep things running. I never gave up the show completely. If I was gone for two or three months, I might as well just resign and forget the years I'd put into *Big Boy's Neighborhood*.

Dr. Quilici explained that he needed to run a catheter into my body so that he could pump in the high levels of protein and nutrients I needed to recover, the ones I'd never be able to take in just through eating alone. This catheter needed to be attached to me, constantly, for several months.

"There's no way I could be off the air for that long," I said.

"Okay, well, you can get a nurse," he said. "You're going to have to wear a backpack that will pump your protein and nutrients into you until your levels get back to where they need to be. It works continuously for twenty-four hours, because you can't eat like that. Even so, this is going to take awhile."

That sounded serious.

"It's a small procedure," Dr. Quilici said, trying to reassure me. "The nurse will come to your house twice a day."

But I wasn't reassured.

All I could think of was the lady with the accent.

But at least Dr. Quilici seemed to think he could help me. I decided to put my faith in him. We reached a compromise.

I went into the hospital. Sure enough, two weeks after meeting that lady, I was on a feeding tube, too. When they released me, I wore a special backpack at all times. It contained a reservoir of proteins and nutrients, which a motorized mechanism pumped directly into my chest through a catheter that looked like an iPod's ear bud. It had to be flushed down twice a day.

I couldn't do anything or go anywhere. If the catheter cord snapped, I only had thirty minutes to get to a hospital and have it reattached. During this time, I had a high risk of experiencing a violent seizure because of the disturbance it would cause to my metabolism and the effects that would have on my blood's plasma levels. If I did have to travel for POWER, a nurse went with me at all times. I was constantly in and out of the hospital, getting more tests. Even when I was out and about in the world, I was under the supervised care of my doctor and my nurse.

During this time, I wanted to talk to the lady I had met and hear what else I should expect. Only, I couldn't find her number anywhere. I went on the air and sent her a shout out, asking her to call the station. Nothing. Finally, I went back to the store where I'd met her and approached the security guard who had introduced us.

"Hey, man, how's she doing?" I asked.

"Oh, she died," he said.

That hit me hard. She had done everything she possibly could to save herself; still, she had died. I walked out of the store. Again, I called Veronica.

"Baby, the lady that had the same problems as me," I said. "She died."

Neither of us said what we were both afraid of: I could be next.

31

BIG BOY'S BACKSTAGE BREAKFAST
WITH J. LO

I wasn't dying, though. Under Dr. Quilici's new plan, it actually seemed like I was getting better. After a few weeks, I wasn't exactly turning around, but my swelling had gone down. I could see that the backpack was doing its job. But my situation was still very risky, especially if anything caused my feeding tube to be severed, as I'd been warned. I was still in and out of the hospital for tests and regular monitoring of my levels.

Right at this time, in April 2005, we had a big event planned with Jennifer Lopez, whose album, *Rebirth,* had just come out. Jennifer had always been a friend to *Big Boy's Neighborhood.* But given her crazy schedule, it took Jason more than a year to finalize her commitment to be part of one of our high-profile promotional events called "Big Boy's Backstage Breakfast."

Once we got Jennifer locked in, we promoted the event for weeks and weeks on the air. We built buzz and gave away tickets until we had seven hundred fans that were pumped up to be there with Jennifer and my crew and me at the breakfast. The only problem was, when it came time for the big day, I was in the hospital.

Now, I'd already been on the backpack for nearly two months, which was long enough for me to know how to take care of myself with it. The people in my life knew I was going through some stuff that meant they couldn't play around with me too much because I was fragile. I'd hosted some POWER events where people had yanked my backpack, thinking they were clowning, not knowing they could have severed my tube and cost me my life. After that, I'd gotten into the habit of making an announcement to the crowd, explaining what my backpack was and why people needed to be careful around it. Given all of that, I figured that on the day of the Backstage Breakfast, I could leave the hospital for a few hours, go interview Jennifer and get myself back into my hospital bed without any problems.

Well, there was one problem: Dr. Quilici refused to check me out of the hospital.

"You can sign yourself out," he said. "There's no way I can stop you from doing that. But as your doctor, I advise you not to."

I heard that, but not really.

How bad could it be? I thought.

I figured I could lie in a hospital bed for five hours, or I could get myself over to Whittier, CA and do this Backstage Breakfast in the same amount of time. Nothing was going to happen. So I called my guys and told them what was going on. They were concerned, but they knew me. I wasn't backing down.

"When you get here, we'll get you right on," Jason said. "We'll do what we have to do. You'll do the interview. And you can get right out of here."

Normally, when we did a backstage breakfast, I was the last person to leave because I signed every autograph and took every picture. This time it would have to be different: in-and-out style.

"Okay, cool," I said.

As I signed my discharge papers to check myself out of Providence Saint Joseph Medical Center in Burbank, I saw Dr. Quilici one last time.

"I'll come back," I promised.

He looked at me with an expression that said: *You're a fool.*

"You know I can't tell you anything, my friend," Dr. Quilici said.

I drove myself to the venue in Whittier and went to find Jason. I was wearing my backpack. As I walked in, I tore off my hospital bracelet and hid my IV line under my sleeve. I had an obligation and I was sure I could pull it off. All I had to do was get through these next few hours. At that time in my life, after things had been so bad for so long, I was in the habit of pulling things off.

I could pull this off, too.

I briefed my crew again on the deal. They knew about the backpack, but when they heard how serious the consequences would be if something went wrong that day, the collective reaction from Liz, Fuzzy, E-Man and QDeezy was, *Whoa!*

We'd been through a lot in the past few months, and we'd get through this, too. The venue was packed with seven hundred pumped fans, who also got the rundown on the backpack, just so everyone would know to be careful of me. Jennifer was waiting in the wings. There was a long table set up in the spotlight. My crew took the stage and waited for me. All I had to do was get up there, take my seat and do my thing.

I walked onto the stage.

People started snapping pictures. This sound went up from the crowd, *Ahh*.

I walked over, kissed Liz, got my headphones on, and we were ready to plug in and play. I pulled my seat out and went to sit down.

As soon as I did, *BOOM*.

I looked down at my chest and saw this white fluid going everywhere.

Oh shit!

When I pulled out my chair, the metal had severed my feeding cord. Now, one end was in my chest, attached to the still-whirring backpack, and one end was just dangling there, with the protein solution I needed to keep me alive flowing out. I picked up that end, and I could see there was no hope of fixing the backpack myself. It was like I had chopped a garden hose in half and there was no way I was putting the two pieces back together. To be repaired, it needed real medical professionals.

The crowd was still cheering. No one had any idea what was going on. But everyone in my crew knew that if my backpack wasn't repaired in the next thirty minutes, I could end up on the ground having violent seizures. I could end up dead.

"Man, Big, we've got to get you out of here!" they said. "We've got to cancel! You've got to go!"

But I wasn't about to give up just like that.

"Dude, just call my doctor," I said.

I took off my backpack and turned off the pump, so at least the fluid stopped flying everywhere. All I could hear in my head was: thirty minutes, thirty minutes, thirty minutes. They had to pull Dr. Quilici out of surgery, but he got on the phone with me right away. I told him what had happened.

"Where are you?" he asked.

"I'm in Whittier," I said.

"How long is the broadcast?" he asked.

"It's probably gonna be about two hours, three hours at the top," I said.

"Okay, my friend, you can do it," he said. "I advise you to leave, but you can make it. If you start to feel lightheaded, you should leave as soon as possible. Turn the machine off, take in lots of fluids . . . ."

He hadn't exactly given me his approval, but it didn't sound like he thought I was going to die, either. Somehow, I just had this feeling that nothing was going to happen to me. So I decided to stay there and keep broadcasting. Of course, this was no small thing. Even Jennifer was freaking out. Someone backstage had tipped her off about the backpack and my critical condition. Just before she was supposed to come out to be interviewed and play a few songs of the album, she pulled me aside.

"We can reschedule," she said. "We really can. I would do it for you, Big."

But I knew that rescheduling would never happen. I shook my head.

"What are you doing here?" she asked. "Get yourself to the hospital!"

"No, I'm fine," I said. "I'm fine."

I was scared. But I also knew how much I could take. I'd physically been through so much already since my surgery that this almost felt like nothing.

Once I got back out on the stage, and Jennifer came out with me, my adrenaline kicked in. I totally forgot about the thirty-minute seizure warning, or the few hours of wiggle room that Dr. Quilici had given me beyond that.

During the whole show, it honestly never dawned on me to even glance at the clock. The next thing I knew, I looked up and it was two and a half hours later, and we were done. That whole time, I hadn't felt sick or lightheaded. There was so much energy on that stage and in that room, and I was having so much fun with Jennifer, my crew and the listeners that the time just flew by.

Of course, as soon as I signed off at the end of the broadcast, I knew that I needed to jet. Jennifer had to leave right away, too, but as she hurried out to her car, she stopped to give me one last concerned look.

"Baby, get out of here," she said.

I could tell she was worried. She didn't even know how bad it really was. I just smiled and nodded and watched her car pull out of sight. Jason shook his head.

"You're crazy," he said. "Get out of here."

Again, people offered to drive me, but I was sure I could make it on my own. Well, I knew I couldn't make it *all* the way to my regular hospital in Burbank, so I got Dr. Quilici on the phone again. He told me to stop in at Shriner's Children's Hospital. He'd arrange for a doctor there to help me. I called my nurse, too.

"I'm minute to minute right now," I said. "Can you meet me at Shriner's?"

My nurse met me. Another doctor sterilized my backpack and equipment and put my unit back together. The doctor gave me a quick IV. Then I jumped back in the car. From there, I drove myself back to Saint Joe's and admitted myself into surgery. Dr. Quilici was waiting. He took me into surgery and replaced the catheter in my chest.

I had made it.

The experience left a strong impression on my crew. From then on, they knew that if I took a day off, I am not playing—and they'd better not be either. Even today, when they call in sick to work, they know it had better be for something good.

32

ON STAGE WITH MARIAH

All told, I wore the backpack for about two and a half months. Slowly, I started to see an improvement and to feel a little bit better. I never did feel great. And it had become clear to me that I'd always be under some kind of medical care for the rest of my life. But the worst of my symptoms had improved: my swelling had gone down. I had more energy.

When Dr. Quilici told me that I didn't need the backpack anymore, I was so happy; but we couldn't start celebrating right away. After my surgery to remove the catheter, he still monitored me closely to make sure that my levels stayed where they needed to be and that I was still feeling alright. Luckily, everything was cool.

After everything I'd been through, I decided to celebrate in a big way when it came time for my next birthday. As I've mentioned, I've always been a huge fan of Ice Cube and Snoop Dogg. I mean, I paid to see those cats so many times, especially Ice Cube. Every year, I do a birthday party, and I'd always wanted to ask Ice Cube to perform. But I'd never done it because I was afraid that he would turn me down.

This time around, I decided to just ask him. Before I had even gotten the whole question out of my mouth, he told me he would do it. I couldn't believe it. He came and did a full show for me, with WC on the mic and Crazy Toones on the turntables, at Club Ibiza in Whittier. We probably had two thousand people packed in there that night.

At one point, I looked up and there he was, my man Ice Cube, on the stage.

"We here for Big Boy," he said. "Big Boy, happy birthday!"

That blew me away right there.

And then, it came time for my favorite part of the set. Ice Cube always does this thing where he walks off the stage and WC calls him on it:

"Fuck you, Ice Cube."

And he comes back out and raps some more.

So they went into that whole bit. Then, just like always, he came back out. He went into the song "The Nigga Ya Love to Hate." I love that record. And he was performing it for my birthday. This was so great. At the end, he started having the crowd give me a shout out. Only it went like this:

"Fuck you, Big Boy!"

Normally, that would have gotten me upset, but that was just amazing, watching this thunderous rapper, Ice Cube, doing all of this for me.

"Fuck you, Big Boy!" he shouted, inciting the crowd.

"Fuck you, Big Boy!" they shouted in unison.

That had always been my favorite part of Ice Cube's show.

That night, it was all for me.

I could have died happy, but luckily, I stayed on the mend. That moment with Ice Cube was probably one of the best I've ever had, in terms of what my position at POWER has allowed me to do in this life. It's just been amazing to go from being the biggest hip hop fan to being a part of the hip hop world and helping to turn on a whole new generation of hip hop fans. Just imagine how I felt when I got to do a show with Kurtis Blow, who was like the original rapper, or the Sugarhill Gang, who I've already given props to as the group that got me into hip hop in the first place.

By this point, I can say I've had all of the big guns in hip hop and R&B on my show, plus plenty of others: Snoop, Ice Cube, P. Diddy, Jay-Z, Eminem, Beyoncé, Mariah Carey, Jennifer Lopez, Janet Jackson, Christina Aguilera, Justin Bieber, Rihanna, Lady Gaga—

even President Barack Obama. We definitely try to see Jennifer Lopez whenever she has a new album or movie out, and always at least once a year. Jennifer is such a good person with *The Neighborhood,* with the crew, and with the audience. We always try to keep her on a rotation. Mariah is always good to pick up the phone and check in, but we try to have her in at least once a year, too. We talk to Beyoncé whenever we can get her.

What's almost as exciting is to have a new artist in for the first time and see that they're trippin' because they can't believe that they're here, or somebody from another city or state who's making it in for the first time. It's like people feel they've accomplished something when they come into *Big Boy's Neighborhood.* That's wild for me. When Flo Rida came through, he gave us props, "Hey, man, I been wanting to get on this show for years."

Of course, there have also been a few people who've wanted to get on the show over the years, but not because they were fans or had the respect. I remember when former Governor Arnold Schwarzenegger came through years ago to promote a movie he'd done. It was before he was governor. He was just about to make the announcement on Leno that he was running. The morning he was due into *The Neighborhood,* I watched through the studio window as he came down the hallway.

What the fuck is Arnold Schwarzenegger doing here? I thought.

My producer, Jason, wanted to do this whole reveal to the audience, make it like a big surprise that Arnold Schwarzenegger was in the 'hood. I was on the air, and Arnold was about to just walk in and blow the whole thing. So Jason put his hands up and went to stop Arnold from entering until I had the chance to do the set up.

Arnold stopped and looked at him.

"Don't touch me with your greasy hands," he said.

Jason stopped short when he heard that, and decided he'd better just let Arnold in, set up or no set up. Well, the rest of his time at *The Neighborhood* was pretty much the same deal. It was clear that Arnold was just here because he was thinking of himself as a politician; he figured he had to do *Big Boy's Neighborhood* because all the stars came through. I wasn't so into that interview. I knew he had never heard of us.

At least Jason and I got a good running joke out of it. We still clown about that to this day: Don't touch me with your greasy hands.

Moments when I've felt disrespected have been rare, but they've stuck with me. I'll bring in anyone and celebrate them. I really will. But I also look at it like, when any star walks in, or calls in, they're coming into my Neighborhood. They're coming into my house. So they're my guests, and I'm going to treat them with respect. But it's the same as if somebody came to my house. I wouldn't let them piss on my sofa.

During everything I'd been through in the wake of my surgery, I hadn't talked about being sick in public, especially not on my show. The way I see it, my job is to entertain people and make their days better, not drag them down with all my problems. I was good at camouflaging what was going on with me. But there had been times when people saw me out in Los Angeles, and there was no denying that something was wrong.

"Why don't you talk about this?" they said.

I knew it probably would have helped ratings or have brought more people in, but I just didn't feel like I needed it. The show wasn't really about that. Sure, the show had been a kind of therapy for me during hard times, but I never wanted that to come across on the air, or for it to seem like a crutch. I worried that people might have started listening differently, like wondering if I was having a bad day, or listening with a sympathetic ear as opposed to a comedic ear. I wanted to entertain.

I always felt like, *Shut up and entertain, you sick bastard.*

But then, in February 2006, I finally went public when I agreed to do an episode of *The Tyra Banks Show*. It wasn't like I'd suddenly decided I wanted to talk about myself. It all happened very organically. I knew the show's producer, Benny Medina, through his role as Mariah Carey and Jennifer Lopez's manager; and he brought me on board for an episode about gastric bypass surgeries.

"Hey, you probably need to tell this story," Benny said.

I respected Benny's opinion. And I remembered how, at my worst, I'd wished that I could find even a single person who knew what I was going through.

"Okay, it's time to talk about it," I agreed.

The show aired on February 15, 2006. The other guests were Carnie Wilson and Jackie Guerra. I've always been glad that I decided to do it. I've had so many people come up to me and tell me that they saw the episode; and I feel like maybe I helped some people to avoid the same problems that I experienced.

This was a good time in my life. Things were going great on *Big Boy's Neighborhood*. Veronica and I were closer than ever. After everything she'd seen me through in the year since I'd undergone my duodenal switch, I knew she was my teammate.

I don't know what I would have done without Veronica. Even though I didn't like anyone to know how bad things had been for me, she knew I couldn't go through all of it alone. She made sure I didn't have to. I later found out that she'd been sending emails to my crew, like: "How's Big feeling? How's he look today? Can you guys remind him to take his proteins?" Of course they're all terrible liars, so I knew that she was getting them to check up on me in some way. That wasn't easy for me. But I knew it was out of love.

And then, we found out Veronica was pregnant. We got ready to start our family. It had been a long haul, but things were finally looking pretty golden.

That October 10, 2006, Mariah Carey was in town for a concert at the Staples Center. The last time Mariah was in town, *Big Boy's Neighborhood* had done two nights with her at the Gibson Amphitheater. This time around, we didn't have anything like that planned, but I did have some plans of my own. I talked to Mariah's manager Benny Medina in advance to set everything up. And then, I went down to the concert to support Mariah and to get a picture at the show for my website. While Veronica and I were backstage talking with Benny, I grabbed Veronica and asked her to help me get the picture I wanted in front of the crowd.

"Baby, I need you to come out and take a picture," I said.

Veronica is real shy about that kind of stuff, so she was trying to hand the camera off to anyone else she could find. But I wasn't having it.

"No, I want you to take the picture," I said.

So I walked out onto the stage. She followed me out there with the camera in her hands. There was a crowd of seventeen thousand people there for the show that night, and as soon as they saw me, they all started cheering, "Big Boy!"

I started playing with the audience; Veronica took a picture for me. Then, before she knew what was going on, I grabbed the mic and got the audience to settle down. As I looked out into the crowd, I could see Eddie Murphy and Magic Johnson amid this sea of faces.

I turned to Veronica and started talking about how special she was to me. She was smiling at me, but I could tell that she wasn't sure what was going on. I think the audience was starting to get it, though, because they got real quiet.

"You're my friend," I said. "The only thing that you're not is—I want you to be my wife."

The crowd went crazy. Veronica was so shocked that she never actually said yes. She just hugged me real big. When I was putting the ring on her, she was shaking so hard that I was about to give up and just put it in her pocket.

I saw the singer Johnny Gill in the crowd, and I pointed at him.

"Johnny, you're going to sing for us at our wedding," I said.

Everybody was cheering and the whole thing was crazy. As we walked back to our car that night, everyone kept shouting at us.

"Congratulations!"

"Congratulations!"

"Congratulations!"

Veronica and I had a lot of happy times to look forward to, but there was just one thing I wanted to take care of first. I had a lot of excess skin from having lost 250 pounds since having my duodenal switch. I hadn't been feeling well enough to exercise and tighten up the flab yet. But even if I had been, this was way beyond what I could have taken care of at the gym.

It wasn't like I wanted to look like Tyson Beckford. I just wanted to have the loose skin removed, which was a really common procedure among people who'd lost as much weight as I had. That excess skin was really starting to become a problem with walking, and bathing, and my day-to-day life. It felt heavy on my frame. It looked crazy. It even sounded crazy.

One time, Veronica and I were in Hawaii, and we were about to take this scenic helicopter ride. This was a new thing for me because I'd always been way over the weight limit for helicopters. I couldn't believe that I actually made the cut. But before we could go, we had to watch an instructional video with some other tourists. As I was walking down the benches to get to my seat, my skin was making this clapping sound. Everyone in the room could hear it, which was embarrassing. Beyond that, the extra skin was annoying. It felt like this constant up and down of extra weight that kind of yanked on me whenever I moved. There were so many health problems that went along with it, too. I ran the risk of infections, frequent boils, and bad circulation. Because the blood couldn't flow as freely as it needed to do, my legs started to swell up again and my stomach got bloated.

Then, just as I was getting on board with the idea of having the surgery, I had a conversation with Ron Lester that actually made me think that maybe it wasn't such a good idea. The way that he was talking about himself, and whether or not this girl or that girl was into him, and whether or not he was going to get this part or that part, really freaked me out. It seemed like all of his self-worth had to do with how he looked. He thought that having the duodenal switch, losing the weight, and then having the skin removal surgery was going to bring him to some kind of perfection that was going to make everything in his life good. I could tell by the way he was talking that he didn't feel any better about himself than he had when he was fat.

Then, Ron lifted up his shirt and showed me his skin removal scars, and I could not believe what I was seeing. He had scars everywhere, so many that his skin looked like a map. I got so freaked out, I ended up having to talk to Jason about it because I didn't know how to wrap my head around what I was feeling.

"No man, that's just him," Jason said. "You're not the same."

Finally, I realized that Jason was right. I had loved myself at 500 pounds. I loved myself now, even with my loose skin. I think that's the key. We all have to do a better job of this in our lives. I'm not saying that you should embrace the fat, because we all know that the fat is going to kill you eventually—and you've got to do something about it. But don't beat yourself up for being fat. Or having some other area of your life that's out of control. It doesn't mean that you're a bad person, or that you don't deserve to be happy. Love who you are, no matter how you look or what's going on in your life. Because if you don't, no matter how much weight you lose, or how many surgeries you get, or how successful you become, or how many goals you reach, nothing is going to fulfill you.

I decided to go ahead and get the skin removal surgery. Our first child was due in early 2007, so I planned the surgery for my 2006 Christmas vacation, in order to be all healed up by the time Veronica gave birth. I figured the duodenal switch and the side effects I'd experienced from that had been the hard part. This was only going to be two or three days in a Beverly Hills clinic. All I had to do was get the skin off, and I'd be a so-called "new" person.

I'd met my surgeon, Dr. Calvert, through *The Tyra Banks Show*. One of the other guests who was on the show with me that day was about to go in for her skin removal surgery, and so her segment was about what was involved. Dr. Calvert was not only her doctor, but he was also supposedly *the* man for this kind of procedure.

When I started talking to Dr. Calvert about my surgery, I probably weighed between 250 and 275 pounds. We agreed that he would cut about 50 pounds of excess skin from my chest and back. At first, I thought that meant I would drop another 50 pounds. But he explained that it didn't quite work like that. After the skin came off, my body would adjust and put some of that weight back on in the places where it needed to be. I still knew the procedure was worth doing.

I wasn't just living in this fantasy land. I knew it was going to be painful. I'm allergic to most pain medications, so I could take an aspirin or a Tylenol, and that's about it.

The procedure involved cutting into a lot of my skin, a common procedure for Dr. Calvert. He kept telling me I'd be in and out. And I took his word. I was ready for the skin to be gone. I was ready to feel and look better. I was ready to see what size shirt I was going to wear afterwards. I was ready for all things positive.

33

ANOTHER BAD DAY

What I wasn't ready for was to wake up in the ICU at Cedars-Sinai Medical Center. But that's exactly what happened after I got the skin removal surgery and fought for my life all the way to the emergency room.

I had made it that far.

That didn't mean the hard part was over, though. The first thing they had to do was stabilize me. I was cut everywhere, just sliced up. This was beyond painful. I was groggy. I couldn't get off the bed. Everybody was poking at me. I was in hell.

At first, I was pissed at Dr. Calvert. I remember he came in, acting all positive.

"We got you through that," he said.

You motherfucker, I thought. *You didn't get me through shit. Dude, you fucking mutilated me. You nearly killed me.*

But as we started to work out what had gone wrong, I knew that it wasn't really Dr. Calvert's fault. The main problem was that I never put Dr. Calvert and Dr. Quilici together. Dr. Calvert didn't know anything about the duodenal switch and how different it was from a regular gastric bypass operation. He had no idea how sensitive my system was. Dr. Quilici knew I was going in for a skin removal procedure but he didn't know the size of what I was getting done. If he had, he would have kicked up my proteins and vitamins beforehand. But because he didn't, and the surgery lasted eight hours, it was too long for my body to be without nutrients. It literally started to grind down on the operating table, just like it had before I got my protein pump.

I was already walking into the surgery half-assed, as far as my health went. Because of that, it hit me so hard that it really just brought me to my knees afterwards. I had nothing to battle back with. I was malnourished. And without the proper nutrients, my blood was so thin that I couldn't clot up right. I didn't get scabs. I just bled. I couldn't heal up from my incisions.

I was releasing blood, and that meant I was losing blood. I had this one terry cloth robe that I wore in the hospital. I wanted to keep it when I was released, but Veronica ended up taking it and throwing it in the trash because it had been soaked in blood while I was in there. I had to get two transfusions—one transfusion of blood and one transfusion of fresh frozen plasma—to help my blood coagulate.

Every day that I woke up in the hospital, I started out by sort of checking in with my body. And every day, my first thought was the same: *Okay, well, it's gonna be another bad day.*

Because I couldn't take any pain medication, I just had to sit up in my bed and wait it out. Those were long days. I couldn't get off the ICU floor until I coughed. They were afraid of pneumonia, or fluid in my lungs, or having my lungs collapse. And so, they wanted to make sure my lungs were strong enough for me to go to a regular room. It took me four days to cough. I literally didn't have the strength.

Finally, I coughed; then I went to a step-down unit, and then I went to a regular room for six days. Even when I was supposedly over the worst of it, my body went haywire. This was another moment when I definitely thought: *What did I do?*

All of the fluid went down to my testicles. They were so swollen and purple that my scrotum looked like an eggplant. I thought that was the way it was going to be for the rest of my life. Fuzzy came to see me, and I just had to show somebody.

"Dude, you've got to see my nuts," I said.

He gave me a funny look, but he knew that after what I'd been through, it must be something crazy for me to even bring it up.

"All right, man, show me," he said.

When I did, he could not believe what he was seeing. It looked ridiculous. I'm not even clowning. Finally, Dr. Quilici had to come up to Cedars and jump in. He helped me to get my levels stabilized and the swelling went down. But it was wild.

After ten days, they finally released me from the hospital. For the ride home, they gave me half of a Percocet, because the pain of being moved would have been too great without it. That felt amazing and was enough to make me realize that my recovery would have been a whole different story if I'd been able to go through all of this on pain pills. But by the time I got to my front door, I was itching so badly that I wanted to scratch my skin off. No painkillers for me.

Even though I was at home, things were still intense for the next two or three months. Every day, when I woke up, the first thing I did was this little crunch up to a seated position. That allowed me to check in with the pain that day, and see where I was at with everything, just like I'd done when I was in the hospital.

Finally, slowly, things started to improve.

Okay, well it's not as bad as yesterday, I thought.

That's how I measured how each day was going to go.

The problem was that I still couldn't heal properly. I had this hole right in my pelvis where they had tightened up all of the loose skin and sewn an incision. It had to be cleaned out regularly and stuffed with gauze. And, sometimes when I coughed, blood and body fluids shot out of the hole. Because I couldn't clot and develop the scab I needed for the wound to heal, my underwear was always full of blood.

I had four drains in me, which were these tubes that were like vacuums in my body. They traveled around inside my body, sucking up extra fluid so my swelling wouldn't be as bad. I had to pull them out and empty them several times a day. When I did, I had to record how much fluid they had gathered. Then, I had to clean them and put them back in. It was just a mess to shower or do anything with them in. I had to have my bandages changed regularly.

Again, I had to have a nurse come to the house to help me with all of this. I had to sleep on the couch with my legs elevated. My protein levels were off. It got scary again. I remember saying to someone during this time:

"I had less problems at 500 pounds than I have today."

This was even worse than when I was depleting after my duodenal switch operation. I had so many moments where I beat myself up, like:

Dude, what have I done? What cost did I pay to be so-called healthy? Couldn't I have just eaten right and gone to the gym?

As badly as I was feeling, I made sure that I wasn't off the air for long. After I got out of the hospital, I did my first few days from the studio at my house. Even that was hard. Everything took so long. When I woke up, I had to empty my drains and clean my incisions. Getting dressed in sweats and a T-shirt was a process because of the drains and how sore and swollen I was. It literally took me two hours to get ready. Finally, I created this thing where I took a shoestring and hung it around my neck, and then I took each drain and used a safety pin to attach it to the shoestring. Once I had that, I was able to get into the shower and that was heaven. Even with all of those drains dangling from around my neck, it didn't even matter. Feeling that hot water on my skin felt so good.

Each step was slow, but each step was a celebration, too. After about three months, I got my drains out. My thoughts changed from that dark place where they had been to: *Okay, I'm going to live. I'm on that road to recovery now.*

Slowly, slowly, things got even better. I was still sore, but I didn't hurt as badly as it had before, so that was huge. My skin started healing up. I could drive again.

Okay, I'm starting to feel normal, I thought.

From there on out, it all felt beautiful. Being able to just jump into the shower without thinking about it was amazing. Being able to go into the studio and see my crew was the greatest. And, best of all, in February of 2007, my son Jayden was born. I finally started to feel like I was well enough to be a dad.

34

MEETING THE KING OF POP

I didn't exactly feel great. But I wasn't at death's door anymore. I could concentrate on my new family and on building *Big Boy's Neighborhood*. We'd been playing with the idea of doing a syndication deal for years. Jason finally made that come together in August 2007 when we signed with ABC Radio Networks. Most of the stations came on board in early 2008. Although we switched our syndication deal to Dial Global Radio Network in 2010, my show is still broadcast in thirty markets. Since the time of our syndication deal, I'm proud to say that not one person has come up to me and said that my show sounds different. That's because I serve POWER and the Los Angeles listeners who have always supported me first; and then, we let the syndication play into what we're doing. It's definitely cool to have a bunch more listeners in all new places around the world.

One of the best things about my job is that I've honestly had the chance to throw down with pretty much all of my idols. But in January 2008, I had the honor of spending time with one of the world's greatest entertainers, MJ. I'd known will.i.am from The Black Eyed Peas since back in the day. During this time, he happened to be in Las Vegas producing a few songs for Michael Jackson, who was putting together the 25th Anniversary edition of *Thriller*. While they were working together, Will told Mike that he should meet me, and Mike told Will to bring me to Vegas. I knew how huge this was. I jumped at the chance.

Will.i.am hooked the whole thing up for us; and Fuzzy stayed on top of it. When the day came, Fuzzy and I got on a plane and flew to Vegas. When we arrived, we checked into our hotel and went straight to the studio where Will and Michael were working at The Palms Casino. After we waited on Michael for a few minutes, I left to go to the bathroom. When I came back, Michael was in the studio with his son, Blanket. I noticed that the light had been softened; there was this nice ambiance, and Michael looked perfect. His hair was done. He was wearing his sunglasses.

"Hey, Big Boy, this is Michael," Will said. "Michael, this is Big Boy."

Mike stood up to greet me, just as polite and pleasant as could be.

"It's a pleasure to meet you," he said.

"Hey, Mike, how are you doing?" I asked.

"That's an awesome shirt," he said.

I looked down. I was wearing a *Big Boy's Neighborhood* shirt.

"Man, Mike, you can have it to tell you the truth," I said.

He started laughing at that, and we just went from there. The whole day was such a good vibe because it was just Michael, will.i.am, one of Will's partners, Peter Lopez, an engineer, Fuzzy, and me. I'm sure there was security around somewhere, but I didn't see them—or even an assistant—at any point in the next three hours. It was very relaxed.

Michael's son, Blanket was in the studio with us for part of the time. Mike was so attentive with him. He really appeared to be such a good Dad, and Blanket was really polite and respectful. At one point, Blanket was trying to get something open.

"Dad," he said.

"Hold on, Blanket, we're talking," Michael said. "What do you need?"

"Can you please open this?" Blanket said.

"Yes, come here," Michael said.

"Thank you," Blanket said.

It was a side of Michael that I had never seen before. It reminded me of how I rolled with my own son, who was about a year old at the time.

While we listened to the songs they were working on, Michael was dancing around the studio with his shades on. We were all just having such a good time. But then, Michael sat down on a studio chair near where I was seated on the couch. We started talking about my POWER billboards. Our conversation got serious.

"How much did you weigh?" Michael asked.

"I was like 510 pounds," I said.

"Oh my God, are you serious?" he said. "What did you eat?"

"Man, Mike, you don't get 500 pounds off of lettuce and tomatoes," I said. "You know that move where you kick your leg up? If I was hungry enough, I would have eaten your leg."

He was just rolling at that. He had a really great sense of humor. It was obvious how much he loved to laugh.

"Wow," he said.

He paused for a second, and I could tell he was really thinking about it.

"Why did you lose the weight?" he asked.

He gave me a look like he really wanted to know. It wasn't just small talk.

"Mike, I was thirty-three at the time, and I did the whole thing of, 'I'm 500 pounds, do I have more time behind me than I actually have in front of me?' You know. You don't really look around and see 500-pound men who live to be sixty-six or sixty-eight. So the answer to my question was that I had more years behind me."

He was looking at me very closely this whole time. He kept nodding his head, really listening. It was like there was nobody else in the room.

"Wow," he said.

Everything I'd heard about Michael being really caring and humorous and fun, I got to experience firsthand during the time we spent together that day.

"So people recognize you everywhere you go?" he said.

"Yeah, people recognize me," I said.

"Can you go to a supermarket and shop?" he asked.

"Yeah, I can go to a supermarket," I said.

"So you can go and actually put things in a basket and push the cart through the aisle?" he asked.

"Yeah, I go shopping all the time," I said. "Who do you think I am, Michael Jackson?"

He laughed at that. But I knew it was a serious question for him, and that he couldn't shop or do anything without getting mobbed.

Like I said, I've met a lot of people, but this was something else. I'm sure Michael had experienced so many conversations like this during his lifetime. Still, it really meant a lot to me to be able to tell him about the impact he'd had on me.

"Mike, man, watching you do the moonwalk on the Motown 25th Anniversary show," I said. "I was thirteen years old, and all of us at school knew that we had just witnessed history."

"Thank you," he said.

It was real gratitude. I could tell by the way he said those two little words.

"It's crazy because, even with *Thriller*, I used to go to my junior high school, and I would practice *Thriller* on the field by myself," I said.

He thought that was hilarious.

"No, dude, I'm serious," I said.

I painted the picture for him of this fat kid out there, all tired and sweaty but still trying to do all the moves.

As we got into talking about *Thriller*, without even realizing it, I had started popping my shoulder. Michael looked over at Peter.

"See, see, what's he doing?" Michael said.

"What am I doing?" I said.

"First thing when you started talking about *Thriller*, you did this," Michael said, and he started popping his shoulder to demonstrate.

Oh shit, I thought. I knew I was seeing something really special right there.

Then we started talking about this SoBe commercial that they were putting together for the Super Bowl, with these lizards doing the *Thriller* dance. Only, in the first version of the commercial, they weren't doing the shoulder pop; as Michael pointed out, the shoulder pop was always the first thing that people thought of when it came to *Thriller*.

"Yeah, you've got to have the shoulder pop in there," Michael said.

And when the SoBe ad did run during the Super Bowl, sure enough, those lizards were doing the shoulder pop too.

At one point, Michael started beat-boxing, and shoulder popping, and moving his shoulders all around. It was like seeing a master at work up close.

During those three hours, I never saw Mike look at his watch or seem like he had somewhere more important to be. The only reason we had to finally leave was because Will had to go do something with Yoko Ono—Michael Jackson and Yoko Ono all in one day. I had to catch a flight back to LA to do the show the next day. So we were off. I felt like Mike and I were planting the seeds to get together again. Maybe he would even come by the show. I didn't ask him for an autograph, which I've regretted ever since. Of course, I didn't know then that we were going to lose him a little more than a year later.

I wasn't going to ask him for a picture either, just because I've always felt weird about that kind of stuff, unless I'm doing it for the show. But, as we were about to leave, Fuzzy brought it up.

"Hey, Mike, can we take some pictures?" Fuzzy asked.

"Oh yeah, yeah, yeah," Mike said.

"Hey, can you take a picture?" I said to Mike.

Mike came over and put his arm around me.

"What are you doing? I said. "I don't want you to get in the picture with me. Who do you think you are, Michael Jackson? I want you to take the picture."

He was laughing so hard. I took the joke further by handing him my camera.

"Oh my God, no one has ever done that to me before," he said.

Mike couldn't figure out how to work the camera. He was almost laughing too hard to take a picture anyhow. After he finally got a picture, I gave the camera to will.i.am to take some more pictures—this time with Mike in them. This was great. Or so I thought. Not to be rude, but when I looked at my camera, he'd taken the most horrible pictures I'd ever seen. I was thinking, *Dude, it's Michael Jackson. Make it good.*

So I grabbed Mike's arm, which was way stronger than I had thought it would be. I could feel his muscles through his shirt.

"Hey, Mike, can you take another picture with me?" I asked.

"Yeah," he said.

I gestured him over to where I was standing.

"Alright, man, come on, let's take the picture," I said.

But I wasn't done clowning yet. Next, I had him pose.

"Mike, I want you to play like we're laughing at something," I said.

That was one picture.

"Let's go back to back, so we're chilling," I said.

We were just laughing and having so much fun.

And then, when it was time to leave, I couldn't believe it: Mike thanked me.

"Thank you," he said. "It was a pleasure to meet you."

I was like: *No, dude, you're Michael Jackson. The pleasure was all mine.*

As soon as Fuzzy and I left Mike in the studio and walked out into the casino, we started losing our minds. I looked around and thought about how, if people knew that Michael Jackson was on the other side of the wall, they would have flipped. I immediately called my family. When I told my sister Sheila, she started to cry.

"Dude, it was off the hook," I said.

"How did he look?" she asked.

"He looked like Michael Jackson," I said.

The whole thing was crazy. Later that day, Peter Lopez called me.

"I just wanted to call you," he said. "Michael really enjoyed hanging out with you today. I'm not calling because he wanted me to call you. But I wanted to tell you that when you were leaving, he was like, 'I know why that guy is a superstar.'"

I couldn't believe Michael Jackson had said that about me. That's exactly what I would have said about him. He was a total superstar and just the nicest person.

I ALSO HAD ONE OF MY BIGGEST all-time professional thrills that year, when I got to interview now President Barack Obama live on-air on two separate occasions. He was a presidential candidate then but I just had such a strong feeling of hope that he would become president. It was so amazing, being able to speak with him and help make people aware of him. One of the calls was when he was campaigning heavily in Pennsylvania. As part of our syndication deal, we were broadcasting on POWER 99 in Philadelphia at the time. It was crucial that he get on the air and speak to people in the state, and so it was such a great thing to be able to help him do that.

Before we went live on the air, I had a minute to ask him how he wanted me to set up my questions, so we could have the greatest impact when I brought him on live. He told me to ask him about the Iraq War and to ask him where people could go vote. He was just keeping it real.

And then, after Obama got elected, I got an even bigger honor when I was invited to the White House for a poetry slam. Fuzzy was the first one who emailed me about it. "Do you want you to go to the White House?"

I hit him back, "Of course I want to go to the White House!"

I had to fly myself out there and get my own hotel room, but of course I didn't care. I was going to see President Barack Obama. And then, we were told that they needed my government name and my social security number for a security check.

I'm not going to the White House, I thought as soon as I heard that.

I mean I've got the kind of marks and blemishes on my record where I figured there was no way they were going to let me in. But I actually got cleared. And that whole trip was such a thrill. I'd been to Washington D.C. before, but never to the White House. My hotel was down the street from it. As soon as I checked in, I walked down there and just took it all in. When we arrived the next day, the security was over-the-top, as you'd expect. Even though I'd had a background check, just to get on the list, we had to go through three or four checkpoints—including metal detectors. Luckily, I didn't have any fat to tuck guns into anymore, so I was cool.

James Earl Jones was there, along with Spike Lee, Vice President Joe Biden, and First Lady Michelle Obama, of course. President Obama spoke. But other than that, it was just kind of a nice, intimate room with people getting up and doing poetry. It really felt like we were at a cocktail party at somebody's house. I didn't feel overwhelmed by the security presence. I had the chance to say hello to the President and shake his hand, which was amazing. Unfortunately, the one shot I had to get a photo with him got messed up and the picture turned out horribly. I guess I have bad luck with photos when it comes to the true greats.

Angie Martinez from HOT 97 in New York City was there too, so I caught up with her. Then, we strolled around together. Walking through the White House was wild! I stuck my head in the theater room and thought about how the First Family really watched their movies in there. It was crazy to see how they really lived in there, like any other family. And, then, just to see all that history was unbelievable. To walk down the hallway and know that all of the presidents at some time had walked down that hallway too, just blew me away. It was great to see the pictures of George Washington and Abraham Lincoln and Bill Clinton. It almost felt like the Clintons still lived there because there were so many photos of Bill and Hillary. That was really special for me, to be this guy who came from the street, and became a radio personality, and got to sit down with the President— and not just any president, but the first African-American president. Not much has topped that.

EVER SINCE I STARTED AT POWER IN 1994, I had been all about the show and the opportunities it brought me, and the things it allowed me to do for my family and friends. When I wasn't on the air, I spent a lot of time alone. I never gave much thought to needing anything more than that in my life or having a family of my own. But ever since I'd met Veronica, my radio career and my personal life had been of equal importance to me. I tried to balance the two as best as I could.

In 2008, I had another once in a lifetime experience that was also one of the happiest days of my life. I married Veronica at our house in Calabasas, CA on June 28, 2008 during a small ceremony in front of eighty of our closest friends and family. In my industry, there are just way too many people; I knew that we were either going to have to do something very big or something very small.

Our music director E-Man had 600 people at his wedding by the time he got done inviting family and industry folk. There are 70-something people just on the floor where we work at POWER. I wanted something where no one would have to introduce themselves to each other.

Our décor was inspired by this birthday party that Benny Medina had at his house, which was in a tent, but was so ritzy that it looked like it was in a private hall. So even though our wedding went down in our backyard—exactly where my basketball court normally is—our guests walked into what looked like a paradise.

We had this cat named Pastor Bobo, who's a minister at my sister's church, marry us. And we hired DJ Rawn, who worked at POWER and is also a great wedding DJ. As for MC duties, there were lots of us there—Fuzzy, Tattoo, and me, just for starters. I ended up just MC'ing the whole thing. I had to have the microphone. At one point, I started singing Johnny Gill's "My My My" to Veronica. I played like my voice was cracking and getting overpowered by another mysterious voice that couldn't be seen. Then, Johnny Gill walked into the tent and sang "My My My" for us from the beginning. It was beautiful. It blew my family and the whole crowd away. George Lopez, who's a good friend of ours, was also there. Benny Medina came through. But other than that, it was low key. It was a great day. I must say, I looked good in my tux, too.

Our second child, a daughter named Jaide, was born on September 24, 2008. With the addition of the little princess, our family is complete. Well, Veronica's been talking so much about getting a dog, so it's bound to happen sooner or later. There has been talk about child number three as well. We'll see about that. I'd be happy to have a bigger family. When I hold my kids now, I look at them and say, "What was I doing before you all got here?"

I know I had a life, but it doesn't even seem real compared to how my family is everything to me now. But the truth is, I know what I was doing before my kids came along, and I tell them so all of the time.

"Daddy was getting prepared for you," I say.

I always tell my friends who are having their first child that there is nothing you fall in love with faster—no girl, no car, no money, no position, nothing in life. The first time they put that baby in your arms, you think: *I just met this baby, and I would kill or be killed for it.* That's real unconditional love. It happens so quickly.

We're trying to give our kids more of a spiritual direction now. We pray with them at night. But every aspect of our day-to-day life together is so important. It all makes me so happy. My main concern now is making sure I get home and create these memories for my kids. I don't think I could possibly feel more blessed.

35

WHAT'S UP, WILL? IT'S BIG BOY.

Let me tell you, no matter how many of these moments I have with Ice Cube or Michael Jackson or President Obama, when those cats walk in, I'm still in *Damn* mode. When someone like Ice Cube walks into the room, I'm still like, *Damn.* I don't get used to that. And I still don't look at myself like, *Oh, man, these are my peers.*

Of course, I also get some pretty cool opportunities to celebrate my family, thanks to my job. For Veronica's thirtieth birthday in January 2009, I decided to do something special for her. I made her a birthday video that had a few friends on it: Usher, P. Diddy, Ne-Yo, Kanye West, Travis Barker, Busta Rhymes and Robin Thicke. Since I'm still a fan first, I felt like: *Wow, they did that for me.*

I think the fact that I remain a fan first actually helps my interviews. I think it's the reason that I'm so enthused and intrigued by the people that come to *The Neighborhood*—I always try to think about what a real fan would want to know. And I conduct my interviews as if you walked in from the street and wanted to ask your favorite rapper some questions. Of course, I do it with a little more flare, but I do it from the angle of still being a fan. I'm not just here for me. I'm here for the listeners; and the listeners want to have that moment of feeling like Big Boy is representing them.

The only time my approach has gotten tricky is when being Big Boy has given me personal access to private moments. I've had to decide if they were meant for public consumption or not. For example, in 2009, I was at Magic Johnson's 50th birthday. First of all, I spent most of my time there waiting for somebody to pinch me and wake me up, or throw me out. But then, I started wondering how much I should share on the air about being there. When I did my next show, I mentioned that I had gone to Magic's birthday party, but I didn't get into what happened. And then, I wished later that I had been more open because I knew how powerful the message would have been for listeners. There was this moment that day when Magic got up and did a prayer. In his speech, he talked about the doctors who had told him that he wasn't going to make it to this birthday party. Not only was that a real moment to witness, but I also think it said so much about the positive example that Magic can be for all of us, and about how we need to be strong—for ourselves and for our families—and do the so-called impossible sometimes.

Walking that line between being Big Boy of POWER 106 and living moments of my life in a more private way is something that I've had to think about more and more in recent years. I'm telling you, I'll sit at my house sometimes and go through my phone. And, for real, I'll look at celebrities' phone numbers and wonder what the hell they're doing in there. Or, I'll have moments where I'm pinching myself—having a great half hour phone conversation, talking some real shit with Usher, or having somebody like Snoop Dog ask if I can come by the studio to listen to what he's recording and let him know if he's on the right path. When I get with cats like that, and I realize that my word means something to them—that's some next level shit. At the same time, those moments aren't equivalent to the moments when I have these same cats in the studio with me, when we've both got microphones in front of us. I get that there's a line between public and private. I certainly have one in my own life.

As much as I love hip hop and respect the greats that I've had the chance to hang with because of my role in the scene, there is one relationship that continues to mean even more to me. And I had a chance to reconnect with this guy recently. Not that long ago, I was at *The Karate Kid* premiere with my family, and I saw Will Smith. I wasn't going to say anything to him because he was with his people, and there was a crowd around him asking for pictures. I don't really like hitting people up during situations like that. But Veronica wanted me to make sure that our son got his picture with Will. So, I finally went up to him.

"Will," I said. "Hey, man, how you doing?"

"Hey, how you doing, brother?" he said.

He was smiling at me, but I could tell he had no idea who I was.

"What's up, Will?" I said, "It's Big Boy."

"Oh sh—" he said, catching himself because he had people around him.

"Oh, damn," he finally said. "What's up, Skinny?"

"Man, it's so crazy," I said. "My wife was just telling me that I lost so much weight that people don't recognize me."

"I did not recognize you," he said.

At first we were just clowning and laughing; then I got serious and started telling him that I was writing a book. I wanted him to be involved.

"I would love for you to be a part of this book," I said, "Because you were very instrumental in what you're looking at right now."

His expression almost made everything I'd been through worthwhile. It meant so much to me that he'd been one of the only people who had the courage to talk to me about my weight when I was at my biggest. I knew that everything he had done for me was sincere. Even crazier, this was the same Will Smith who I'd first had my picture taken with at that rap conference back when I was only nineteen years old and trying to make it as an MC. Not only had Will been there for some of the biggest moments of my life, he'd literally helped save my life.

Knowing people like Will, who have been around for every incarnation of Big Boy, is even more special these days, now that some folks don't know the *bigger,* old Big Boy anymore. I recently had some teenaged Justin Bieber fans visit me in the studio.

"Why do they call you Big Boy?" one of the girls asked me.

I pointed at some pictures of the billboards that we have in the studio.

"That's me," I said.

"No, it's not!" she said.

"No!" her friend said.

They were shrieking in that way that only fifteen-year-old Justin Bieber fans can shriek.

"How did you lose all that weight?" she said.

So I told them the whole story. Every word was true, but it still felt crazy.

Not as wild as what one of the women I work with at POWER said to me not that long ago, "I never worked with Big Boy."

I may not look like Big Boy, but I'm still Big Boy.

I know I've lost a lot of weight, though. There are so many ways I can tell. I'm reminded when I step on a scale, in how my clothes fit now, when I fly on an airplane and I can buckle my seatbelt without an extension. But one day, not that long ago, it hit me how I really knew: Kids don't call me fat anymore. Kids are the most truthful human beings on the earth, and so I used to hear it from them all the time:

"Mommy, look at that fat man."

Those moments did not feel good. Did they make me run out and eat an extra large pepperoni pizza to dull the pain? Not quite. I think it's a lot more complicated than that, but they definitely contributed to a whole approach to food that was pretty unhealthy. And now, those moments are gone from my life. That's one of the main reasons I've wanted to share my story. I've seen that it's possible to change for the better—that it allows you to live on a whole new level when you upgrade your life. And, think about it, I did it the hard way. I denied that I needed to change. Then I let myself think that it was impossible to change for so long that I ended up needing a lot of help to change. Even when I did finally make a change, I was still in denial about the root of my overeating and how it was playing out in my life. It almost didn't turn out so good for me. But you don't have to let it get to that point. You can start today and make any kind of improvement in your life that you want to make. Even if you don't have everything totally under control, or understand everything about the things in your life that you need to change, you can still take small steps every day to improve your health, your well-being and your life. Believe me, it's worth it. And there's nothing to be afraid of—you'll still be you, only better.

Like I said, no matter how much weight I've lost, I'm still Big Boy. And I'm still bringing it. Really, the amazing moments in my life don't ever stop.

On November 24, 2010, I did something that I've been vowing to do for years. There's this huge, iconic Latino singer Vicente Fernandez who is a god in Latino culture—as he should be. I mean when this man passes, the Latin world is going to shake. Whenever he comes to Los Angeles, he sells out nine nights at the Gibson Amphitheater. Easily. We've always had a good relationship. Every year, he does our show; or I go support his concerts.

Well, Vicente has this song that I just love called, "Aca Entre Nos." And for probably eight years, I've always said that, someday, I would get up with him and sing that song. Finally, last year I told him about my dream.

"I want to sing that song onstage," I said.

"If you're going to sing it, you've got to sing it all in Spanish," he said.

"Alright," I said.

I knew if this went bad, it could have had me run out of L.A. Still, I took the challenge. I deadlined myself by talking about it on the air and having him announce it to his fans. There was no going back after that. Not that I didn't think about it.

It didn't help that everyone was talking about it. I would go places and people would approach me about it, "Man, you're getting on with Chente?"

Gulp.

But I had said I would do it, so I was going to do it.

Veronica is fluent in Spanish. I didn't want to make her listen to me butchering the words until I had them down. I have a partner by the name of Jose who works with this singer Nacho. So they made a CD for me that was just the instrumental track of the song. They also made me a CD of Nacho singing the song, but slowed down, so I could really hear the words. Together, we wrote them out phonetically. For weeks, I drove around and listened to Nacho sing the song. And then, when I was comfortable enough, I recorded myself singing the words over the instrumental section. Then I drove listening to that.

Finally, it was the day of the show. I got a suit like Vicente wears, a big sombrero, the whole outfit. Now, there was *really* no going back. And there was no messing up either. I mean I wasn't clowning. This man is a legend, and I was up there with all respect. To add to my nerves, I never rehearsed with the band until just before the show, and only had just enough time to go through the song once.

Then, it was my moment in the spotlight. During his regular show, Vicente announced me. I stepped onto the stage. I just nailed it. That was the best feeling. People still come up to me and tell me that I did a great job that night.

I would never do it again. But that was a bucket list moment for me. Now I can cross it off.

I had another big moment on *The Neighborhood* not that long ago. Back when I was bodyguarding for the Pharcyde, it was a great hip hop moment because groups like them, De La Soul and A Tribe Called Quest had the world's ears while pushing the boundaries of what hip hop could be. Well, in July 2011, Tribe dropped a documentary, *Beats, Rhymes & Life: The Travels of A Tribe Called Quest* that included a lot of the bullshit they were going through as a group at the time when they were in the prime of their music career. Now, even though I'd been a fan back then, I didn't know the size of it in terms of how they couldn't get along until I saw this movie. As I watched this documentary, it was just crazy to see what they were going through, especially because I had loved them so much for so long. Before the movie was released, we decided to do something on it for the show. Q-Tip wasn't doing any press for the movie, but in June when I had Phife Dawg on the show, we called Q-Tip, and he actually talked for a bit.

It was one of those moments. It was like you could still hear the hurt in their voices. You could still hear the fact that they needed to build in order to get to the point where they could perform or do something together again. There were absolutely no promises made on the air that day, but we still got the conversation started. To be able to have that happen on my show was affirming. It wasn't like I felt that I struck one for hip hop or anything like that. But it was like, *Damn, this interview isn't happening anywhere else.* I think the only reason it did happen on my show is because of how comfortable they were with me after all of these years. That was a huge honor for me, as a fan, first and foremost.

Sometimes the interviews I like doing the most are more about personality than hip hop. I have to say that I still really enjoy having Simon Cowell on the show. He appears so intimidating on *American Idol*. To see him drop his guard and have a good time, it's always funny as hell. Just getting that guy laughing is the best thing. He has this crazy hysterical laugh. It's so fun and high energy whenever he's here. I think he really gets my wit; there are times when he's on the show, and he'll just double over laughing. That's one of the best moments for me.

The other moments I value the most are when I run into listeners, a.k.a. *Neighbors*. I still trip off the fact that people want to take pictures with me or have me sign something for them or tell me that they remember meeting me ten years ago or that they were listening to POWER when I announced that Tupac died. Even my wife, when we first started dating, she found an autograph that I had given her when she was fifteen. She had kept it for all those years. That shit is crazy to me.

It makes me remember back in my day when it was Russ Parr at KDAY that was the main cat for hip hop in Los Angeles. It's wild to think that I could be anything like that for hip hop fans in Los Angeles today. And not just in L.A., either. I've had cats come up to me in South Africa. It's off the hook when I go to Japan, so much so that I do appearances over there several times a year.

I honestly feel like I've done a lot of my bucket list items at this point in my life. I can say that I'm happy with where I'm at with *Big Boy's Neighborhood*. It has been a little crazy for the last couple years, though. Just as I was getting this book ready, we had to let Tattoo go from the show in July 2010. I love Tatt. We had a lot of great years together. I'm sure we'll work together again. Maybe not at POWER, but somewhere, maybe on the radio or on TV. I can say that he is a hell of a personality, and I know there's no replacing that dude. Every day in the studio, there were things coming out of his mouth that I just couldn't believe. If someone had written those lines for him, it would have sounded fake and nobody would have believed it. All we had to do was turn on the mic and—*BOOM*—it was just there. It was just genius.

And then, in August 2011, Liz's time on the show came to an end. Liz was another one who was just a dynamite talent. I used to call her

Sunshine because she had this amazing energy. She was always great to be around in the room. I know she will continue be deeply missed around the studio, and she will always be a part of my life. I couldn't have been happier when I heard that she signed a contract with E! Entertainment Television, and I know she'll have a long and successful career.

But it was time for a change. I can predict that the show is going to continue to change. Radio is different today than it was when I started out. It has a different place in our culture than it did. I can't tell you how many times I've had 50 Cent or someone come in, or call in, and record something with me for broadcast on *The Neighborhood* the next day. Then, by later that same night, before we've had a chance to use it, the audio is dead. Maybe he called into another show in between, or something got released on the Internet and went viral.

If *The Neighborhood's* not always going to be the first place for hip hop fans to get their news, then we have to start thinking about it being something else for them. Not only that, but every three or four years, the audience's palate changes. We need to change too, just to keep things new. So we're always throwing things up against the wall to see what works. The last thing we ever want to do is to make personnel changes, but sometimes it needs to happen.

I can say, though, that the cats backing me at *The Neighborhood* are a great supporting cast, and not just in the case of radio. They're a great supporting cast in my life. Radio is what we do, but afterwards, if I need to talk to somebody—and not just about the show—I call the people I work with because they're my friends.

I'll always keep it fresh and keep it real for my listeners on the air, but I don't feel like I have to sweat it as much after seventeen years on this job. That allows me to start thinking about other ventures. Recently, I did some stuff for my good friend George Lopez on his television show before it was canceled. I've also got a few TV projects of my own in the works.

I feel so blessed to have all of these opportunities. I love to work, but I'm really at my happiest when I'm home with my family these days.

Right now, my main priority, besides my family, is stabilizing my health. For a long time I was thinking about getting the skin removal surgery done on my arms and legs, but I've come to the point where I think I might leave everything as it is now. I mean, when I got the skin from my chest and stomach removed, it almost killed me. I know that I'd go into it educated now. But, even still, I have to question if it would be worth it, given that I struggle on a good day just to feel normal. I probably always will.

On the worst days, I used to wonder if I'd made a terrible mistake by having the duodenal switch, and if I'd actually taken years off my life. Unfortunately, I've had some of these dark days recently, but I do feel like the surgery was the best decision for me overall. For a few years, it had seemed like my levels—which refer to the amount of protein and vitamins I have in my system—had stabilized, and I thought I was making my comeback. But the whole of 2011 has been rough for me: swelling like crazy, and never being able to keep my health where it needs to be. Dr. Quilici has even been saying that I may need to get the backpack put on me again. We've even talked about reversing the procedure, which a few doctors are just starting to do now, even though it was once considered irreversible. That's not an easy decision for me because I've been post-duodenal switch for eight years now. I'm used to being able to eat some of the things I shouldn't be eating, and having my body help kick out some of the fat. Once my body is allowed to absorb the nutrients I need to be healthier, it will also absorb fat, and I'll have to pay more attention to what I'm eating and stay active; if I'm not watchful, I could gain a little weight. But if that has to happen for me to be healthier and feel better, so be it.

36

CLOSE TO PERFECT

Sometimes I feel like a poster child for gastric bypass. Ever since I had my surgery, I've had hundreds of people come up to me and ask me about it, or tell me about how they're going to get a surgery done themselves. If it doesn't happen once today, it'll happen twice tomorrow. I'm always happy to stop and talk to people.

I know how hard this stuff is. Getting real with myself, and changing my approach to life in order to get my weight in check, is the hardest thing I've ever done. But I didn't have a choice. If I hadn't done it, I would have died. This is serious for all of us. One-third of the U.S. population is considered obese by medical standards these days. Michelle Obama has called the obesity epidemic "unacceptable." African-Americans and Latinos are having the most severe problems of all. Bad eating habits, lack of education, and denial are killing our community. We've got to band together and tackle this head on. Nothing else will do it.

As we know, being fat doesn't have a social stigma in the African-American and Latino communities. And while that's good—because I don't want anyone to feel badly about themselves because of their size—being okay with being fat is a huge part of our denial. Look at how it contributed to my own weight problems throughout my life, along with the fact that I wasn't willing to admit that there was an emotional layer to my compulsive overeating. It's time to end the denial and get real about making changes that can save our lives. I paid dearly for my tuition to the school of experience, but I hope you won't have to. I know that everybody comes around when they come around, but maybe my story can be one thing that finally helps you make a change and improve your life.

I do feel like I have a responsibility to share my experiences and what I've learned from them. I'm disturbed because I see some people who are so casual about getting surgery. It's like, as a culture, we've got this vending machine of weight loss surgeries. People think they can just pop a quarter in and pick a surgery, like they'd pick a snack. Only when they push this button, they'll be skinny.

What concerns me is that more and more people seem to see surgery as a solution without understanding what it is. Surgery is really just a tool. The same as diets and exercise are tools. What I've found is that these tools can only do so much. The most important thing is how we use them as part of a larger shift in our consciousness about the way that we live. There's no diet, surgery, or one change in life that's a cure-all. Anything you struggle with: weight, smoking, shopping, or letting people in our lives walk all over us, is not going to resolve itself overnight. The attitudes and issues inside of us that drive this behavior aren't just going to go away. But if we get real about our issues, we can make lasting improvements, especially when it comes to our health.

The best advice I can give is to try to take better care of yourself. Do as much as you can on your own. Hit the gym. Eat right. If you don't already know how, find out. Start making better choices about how and what you eat. Let the people who care about you get real with you about your weight and what it's doing to you, like Will Smith did for me. And then, if you feel like you can't lose the weight on your own, and you need help like I did, do as much research as you possibly can. Read up on surgery, talk to people, go to meetings or classes, take the psych evaluation and give yourself some time to really think about it before deciding on any surgery.

I'm the first to admit that a huge part of making any health plan work has to do with taking responsibility to make sure you eat right, which I don't always do. Clearly this was a problem for me when I was 500-plus pounds. So—no surprise—it's still a problem for me now. Even to this day, I still cook and shop a certain way, which almost always involves buying and preparing more food than I or my family needs. If you look in my refrigerator right now, you will see leftovers. And I'm not saying leftovers are a bad thing. But I'm saying that, in my case, they're not just leftovers. They symbolize something larger. Call it a food addiction, call it a compulsion; there's a part of me that doesn't know what's "normal" when it comes to food. I have to watch myself all of the time. The truth is that I'm not always great at this.

I still eat more than I should, and I have a hard time saying no. I've watched Jason when we're at the studio. He'll be offered something to eat, and he won't take it. That's still hard for me to do. Not long ago, Tattoo offered me some chicken. I tried to be good. I wasn't even hungry.

"Man, I just ate," I said.

"Oh, man, just take it," he said.

"If I don't turn down something, I'll eat everything," I said.

I'm still working on my relationship with food. I know that I'm supposed to have 125 grams of protein a day, and yet, sometimes I'll still eat spaghetti for dinner, just because that's what I want. Then when I start to feel badly, or my hands start to cramp up, I know that's what comes with not doing what I'm supposed to do. And I'll try to tell myself that I can double up on my protein tomorrow. Well, there's no doubling up with this. When I don't take care of myself, there are consequences. They can be worse than you think.

Obviously, I'm an extreme case because of my surgery, but the truth is that you and your body aren't any different. What I've learned is that we need to listen to our bodies. My body just happens to talk back a little louder than yours, but yours is talking to you, too. Pay attention to when you feel hungry, and even more importantly, when you feel full. Work towards only eating when you're hungry, stopping when you're full. Don't eat again until you're hungry. I know this sounds like kindergarten stuff. But some of us need to go back that far because that's when our bad habits started. Don't expect any change to happen instantly.

Once you've pinpointed a few healthy foods that you enjoy and that agree with your body, pay attention to how you feel when you eat them, as opposed to how you feel when you eat the bad foods you love, like pizza and fried chicken. The truth is that healthy food makes your body feel better. I think we sometimes just get used to feeling so badly all of the time that we don't make these basic connections anymore.

I happen to be fortunate enough to have a nutritionist to help me stay on point. Anyone who has a weight-loss surgery will be given a nutritionist, too. But in order for this to be any good, you've got to actually be open to learning from your nutritionist. Truth is, I never really consulted my nutritionist like I should have. Now that I'm older, and I've come so close to dying, I'm better about it because I'm really thinking about getting as many years out of this body as I can.

I'm forcing myself to stop eating several hours before I go to bed so that I don't go to sleep with food in my system. I'm learning to push myself away from the table after I've eaten a reasonable portion. I'm learning to say no to food when I'm not hungry. Hardest of all, I'm admitting that I can't eat the foods I once loved—fried chicken, mac and cheese and red beans and rice—like I once did. They're a special treat now. They're not the foods I turn to on a daily basis. When I do reach for something not so great, say at the studio, I immediately give half of it away. Because I know that, otherwise, I'm going to eat it all. I'm training myself to choose energy food and healthy snacks. I'm watching out for the portion distortion that all of us grew up with here in America. It's crazy because, when I travel to Japan, I'd have to order two or three plates of food to equal what's considered a single portion at a restaurant here. And that gets inside of our heads. When I go out to eat, I still fight the urge to order food with the mentality I had when I was at my biggest.

One of the best things that I've done for my health is to team up with my wife and my crew to make it easier for all of us to eat and live right. We're trying to establish good habits in our house. I still find myself hanging around my kitchen more than I should and cooking food that we don't need. Now that I'm raising kids, I have more of a reason to be aware of how I handle food more than ever before—and not just because I want to stay healthy and be around for a long time with them, either. I know that if I'm not careful, I can put my habits in them. I don't want them to go through any of what I've been through. My wife already says that she can see how much our daughter Jaide is like me. She's not even three. But she loves food. She'll eat anything. She'd eat a piece of brick and think it tasted good.

So, Veronica and I know that we have to be careful about the food that's in the house. We've got to be careful about how we act around food. We've got to be careful about not using fast food as a reward. It's not easy. But it's worth it. It's love. We don't reward our kids with cookies. Usually, we try not to even have cookies in the house. When we have parties, we make sure the extra food leaves the house immediately afterwards so it's not left around as a temptation.

What we do always have around is fresh fruit that's already cut up, and tomatoes and carrot sticks. That way, when my hand-to-mouth habit kicks in, I'm putting healthy food into my mouth, not potato chips or sweets. We cook with healthier oils like olive and grape seed. We try to bake and grill instead of frying. We try not to use butter.

Some of this is stuff that I have learned as an adult, because I wasn't educated properly when I was young. I know a lot of us weren't. But I think we also have to admit that a lot of this is just common sense that we have chosen to ignore. I mean let's get real. We know what makes us fat. Eating too much of the wrong foods. As I've said, I didn't get fat from eating too much lettuce and tomato. I don't have to tell you not to put that much butter on your bread. We know this stuff. We just have to apply what we know.

Again, this is where our family members and our friends can help. My wife is my teammate at home. I've also learned so much from my crew at *The Neighborhood*. We're all trying to get healthier together. Three or four years ago, it was just the opposite. I was putting my bad habits on them and allowing them to enable me with bad habits of their own. I was BBQ'ing and making mac and cheese along with all of that unhealthy soul food that I grew up eating. I was bringing it into the studio with me. We used to grub. And then, I noticed that *The Neighborhood* started gaining weight. Even Liz started gaining weight, and she was usually the one who ordered egg white omelets. That made me really conscious of the impact of food and the impact of community. Now when I go to the store, I buy all of the fresh vegetables that I can find, and I make these beautiful salads. We all eat that instead. Just like I had my eating buddies who used to stop and get a burrito with me after the club, now my crew and I support each other in different, healthier ways. I'm conscious of trying to surround myself with people that can help me to keep my eating in check. It's great to see it paying off for everyone.

My cat DJ Ray used to eat the worst food, like beans cooked in lard, because that's how he grew up, just like me. Now, he's all about egg whites and lean meats, and when he wants a snack, it'll be celery sticks or strawberries. And that means when I'm in the studio with him, and I want a snack, I'm more likely to reach for a piece of his celery, which is good for me, too. When he got serious about eating better, he got a cooler and started bringing healthy food into the studio from home. So I went and got myself a cooler. Now I pack my own healthy meals, too.

Of course I know we're all busy and it's not like we've all got the time or are organized to the point of carrying around coolers of healthy food with us at all times. I still sometimes go to my great childhood love, McDonalds. Only, now, I know there's pretty much nothing for me there. But, when I need something to eat on the go, I can get two or three little salads and throw some raisins and nuts on there. That's a good meal for me. I'm not trying to claim that I never get a burger from McDonald's, either. Like I said, I still let myself have treats on some days.

But the truth is that it's hard to go back and forth. If I'm eating the fatty, rich food that I've always loved, that's what my palate's primed for, and that salad is going to taste bland. But once I've eaten right for two or three days, my appetite drops, my palate changes. When I get into seafood and salad mode, I can really taste everything in that salad. If I'm on point with my eating program, that salad is just a burst of flavor. I know those treats are a trigger for falling off program. I have done it so many times in my life, and had so many Mondays when I've had to start over. I'm trying not to do that anymore.

That said, there are times when I push it. If I eat too much, I throw up. I know this, and yet I've pushed it again and again. At one point, I was throwing up every day. I knew this was disgusting and bad for me—it burned my esophagus and took the enamel off my teeth—and yet I couldn't stop.

Sometimes, I know I shouldn't eat something, and I eat it anyway, and just kind of chance it. I had to build my system back up to drink milk after my surgery, and there are times when I know I shouldn't eat ice cream, but I do anyhow. I haven't totally resolved my relationship with food, but I'm not giving up. I am a work in progress. I'm going to be under construction forever.

That's a major part of my message. Any of the mental stuff—whether it's emotional eating, or what I think was behind my eating, which was just a real addictive or compulsive relationship to food—will still be inside of you, even if you get weight-loss surgery or try every diet out there. Some people think it's going to be a cure-all, but it's just not so. The surgery is not going to do anything to fix any of your habits or behaviors. That's true of how you feel about yourself and your body too. Like I said, I always had a hard time talking with Ron Lester about his procedure because it bummed me out how he thought it was going to make him this happy person who had this life he'd always wanted—getting the big movie roles and the hot girls. I hate to break it to you, but life doesn't work that way. I think he's found that out the hard way because, like so many people who have had surgeries, he's gained some weight back. He's not fat, but I can see that in his own mind, it's almost as if he still is. If you're not mentally strong, and you're not able to find a way to love yourself at any size, you're not going to come out on the other side of a procedure or diet feeling any better than you did when you went in. You may lose the weight, but you'll just replace the fat with some other reason to hate yourself.

So it's time to make a choice. It's time to get real with ourselves and live the best lives that we can—for our families, for our communities, and for ourselves. Let me tell you, you're never going to find perfection. I don't even know what that looks like. But, in my eyes, I'm close to it, just the way I am. And that's where I want all of you to be too. If you can learn to love yourself, and be happy with where you're at, you might already be a lot closer to perfection than you ever thought.

ACKNOWLEDGMENTS

To my beautiful family.

My best friend and rock, Veronica, thank you for being the best wife and the greatest mother. I breathe for you. To my kids, Jayden and Jaide, you make daddy so happy and you are the true reason I get up in the morning. I never knew I could love so much.

Now I know.

To my brothers and sisters, we experienced a lot, and look at us now. Ida raised a beautiful Unit. We were always so affluent in "love." Keith, Charlene, Sheila, Sherrille, Kenneth, and Dr. Nicole, I'm so proud to call you my family.

I will always love and cherish you.

My nephews . . . Ian, Khody, Khoury, and Kyler, I pray my son grows to be just like you gentlemen. Love you truly.

My nieces . . . Caressa, Destiny and Laida, uncle's watching you. No boys 'til you're 50. Love you.

My in-laws . . . Lakisha Alexander, thank you for making my brother, Mouse, so happy. Marko Purifoy, thank you for being the man Charlene deserves. My mother and father-in-law, Ricardo and Hilda Oseguera. Lorena, Gollo, Sara, Adrian, Abraham, Alex, Richard, Stacy, Richie, Cassie and Leah.

The Stapp family.

Thank you for accepting me.

Love you.

Ok, here we go.

To Augie Johnson, thank you for believing in me from the beginning. To The Radio God Rick Dees. Love you. Barry L and Geno. We have many years behind us and plenty in front of us.

To Cupid, love you bro. Let's get you back to 100%.

To Khary Lee, Jason and Eric White, my crew for life.

Mike Carranza. Frank Bonilla.

To Jason Ryan, thank you for being a Super Producer and great friend. We've built a lot and we have a ways to go.

Rick Cummings, thank you for hiring me and hearing something in me that I never knew I possessed. Val Maki, Jimmy Steal, Fernando Lujan, Dianna Jason, and Jeff Smulyan, love you.

To Liz, you have no idea what you mean to me. I cherish our friendship. Keep smiling.

Fuzzy, I love and value you. I love how much you love. You're a great friend. Love you for life.

DJ Ray and Shaun Juan. The architects of "Big Booooooy." Look what we created. Love you. Real friends.

The 'Hood . . . DJ E-Man—dopest DJ in the world, Jeff G., Lalu, Sketch, Rikki, Louie G, Nicky, Krystal B, Joel M., thank you for your hard work.

Joe Grande, QDeezy and Tattoo, you will ALWAYS be a part of BBN. Love y'all.

Yesi—the super woman, Felli Fel, and J. Cruz, keep Power sounding amazing. Power 106 fam, I love each and every one of you.

Flava Unit y'all!!!

Baka Boyz . . . Eric V. amd Nick V. Thank you for putting me in a position to make my dreams a reality. You guys are truly the blueprint for Power 106. Baka baaaayy bay.

Shouts to Ice Cube, WC, Toones, Bro Ron, Mack 10, Snoop, Daz, Kurupt, Soopa Fly, Game, Xzibit, Tha Liks, King Tee, DJ Pooh, Roger Clayton, Egyptian Lover, Mix Master Spade, Toddy T., Greg Mack, Russ Parr, Julio G., B-Real, Sen Dog, Muggs, Bo Bo, Frost, Ice T., M-Walk, Tone Loc, Eazy E, Ren, Yella, Dr. Dre, Coolio, DJ Aladdin. Love to all my West Coast blueprinters.

Baby and Slim Williams. I'm Cash Money now!!! Thanks to all CMC.

To Sarah Tomlinson. Thank You for putting my life into words. You're an amazing person and I enjoyed my "thereapy" with you.

Will Smith: Thanks you for being an inspiration and turning a light on. Love you, big Will.

Evan Weiss and Gary Binkow. We did it.

Jennifer Lopez, thank you for caring. Mariah Carey, thank you for giving me your stage to propose to Veronica. George Lopez, Benny Medina, Diddy, Tyrese, Ne-Yo, Derek Fisher, Magic Johnson, Johnny Gill, Darius Rucker, Jenny Delaney, Fernando Vargas, Steve Harvey, Earthquake, Gabriel Iglesias, Bill Bellamy, Jamie Foxx, Oscar De La Hoya, Mike Tyson, Liz Laud, Natalie Madriz, Sandella, Grady Gaynor, Armida and Tony "Pops" Padilla, Travis Barker, Paul Wall, Skinhead Rob. RIP Lil' Chris. Morrie Sage RIP.

Fred Toczek, get my money.

Min. Tony Muhammad, Bro. Steve, Bro Larry—As Salaam Alaikum. Louis Romo, Ralph Verdugo, Bryan Elms, Preston Williams, Kevin Columbus, Jeff Clanigan and Code Black.

The Pharcyde . . . Imani, Booty Brown, Fatlip and Slim Kid 3. Thank you for the 1st passport stamp and showing me the world. Brothers for life. Paula Stuart, Suave, Syl, Mark Luv, Schmooche Cat, J Swift, Wascals, and Quentin. We experienced a Bizarre Ride!!!

Dr. Quilici, thank you for bringing me back to life.

Dr. Smith, thank you for being a life saver.

Dr. Calvert, bless you for being a great surgeon. Just wish I was a great patient :-)

To The Alonso Unit. Thank you for being a part of my everyday existence. Jose and Jennifer, thank you for the prayers and for always being my highway to more faith.

This book is also dedicated to Christian Anthony Alonso. Gone too soon. One day, we'll be Together In His Arms.

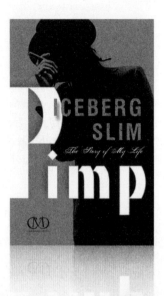
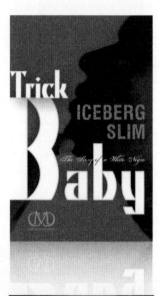
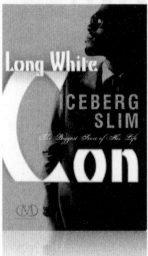
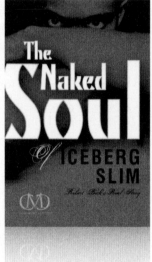

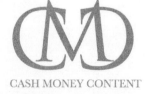

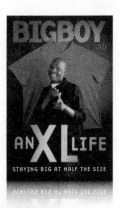
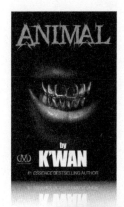
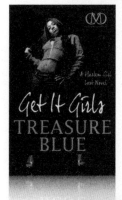
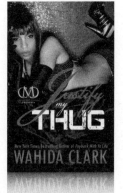
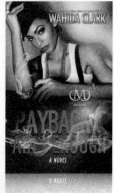
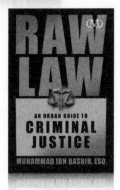
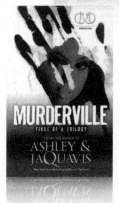

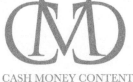